HEALTH CARE POLICY

HEALTH CARE POLICY

A Political Economy Approach

THEODORE R. MARMOR
JON B. CHRISTIANSON

SAGE PUBLICATIONS
Beverly Hills / London / New Delhi

- 1982

For information address:

SAGE Publications, Inc.
275 South Beverly Drive
Beverly Hills, California 90212

SAGE Publications India Pvt. Ltd.
C-236 Defence Colony
New Delhi 110 024, India

SAGE Publications Ltd
28 Banner Street
London EC1Y 8QE, England

Printed in the United States of America

Library of Congress Cataloging in Publication Data

Marmor, Theodore R.
Health care policy.

Includes bibliographies.
1. Medical policy–United States. 2. Medical economics–United States. I. Christianson, Jon B. II. Title. [DNLM: 1. Health policy–United States. 2. Policy making. WA 540 AA1 M35m]
RA395.A3M375 362.1'0973 82-822
ISBN 0-8039-1826-7 AACR2
ISBN 0-8039-1827-5 (pbk.)

FIRST PRINTING

Contents

Acknowledgments

We wish to thank M. Kenneth Bowler, Thomas C. Heagy, Robert T. Kudrle, Walter McClure, James A. Morone, and Donald A. Wittman, who were co-authors of chapters in this book. Chapters 4, 5, and 7 appeared previously in the *Journal of Health Politics, Policy and Law.* Chapter 8 was published in the *Milbank Memorial Fund Quarterly/Health and Society,* and Chapter 6 appeared in the *Journal of Health and Human Services Administration.*

The helpful comments of Terry L. Anderson on an initial draft of the manuscript were most appreciated, as were the considerable efforts of Julie Greenberg in editing various drafts.

—TRM and JBC

Preface

This book results from our shared interest in the formulation and implementation of public policies affecting American medicine. In our separate research we both found a "political-economic" model of explanation most useful in resolving questions of why the United States has developed its current array of policies. This model assumes that politicians, bureaucrats, and consumer-voters pursue primarily their own specifiable interests in the policymaking process. It provides systematic explanations for those instances where the effects of public medical care policy are simply different from stated goals or are clearly contrary to widely accepted notions of what the public interest would warrent.

The political-economic approach to policymaking treats the role of the private marketplace in a similarly unromantic manner. We take for granted that private transactions form the basis of the economic system in the United States. But public sector interventions in this private market also occur, according to the model, largely because they confer benefits on particular groups of individuals. Government intervention does not necessarily have as its objective the correction of a private "market failure," though this rationale may be used as its justification, or may be one of the outcomes of public policy. Both because the "public interest" is not the primary motivation of much government intervention and because public agencies do not operate with perfect efficiency, private mechanisms for the delivery of medical services will not necessarily be "improved" by government actions. If this view is accepted, appropriate public policy requires a comparison of the private market with and without a particular government intervention. Further, it requires recognition that neither the public sector nor the private market is likely to operate as smoothly as its advocates might claim.

While the literature on market imperfections is extensive, the corresponding literature on the operation of the "political marketplace" is not. This book summarizes the more important principles of the political-economic model of medical care and illustrates their applicability to a number of policy topics. Our primary objective is to communicate a realistic picture of policy processes affecting the allocation of medical care. Our intended audience includes students of public policy, particularly medical care policy, those engaged in formulation of medical care policies, and those affected by them.

The book can be read as two separate parts. The first chapter discusses frustrating recent experience with public medical care policies. The second chapter describes the private market for the delivery of medical care, its characteristics, and its potential for producing inefficient and inequitable results. In the third chapter the political processes affecting medical care are described. They too have some undesirable characteristics, many of which parallel the inadequacies of the private market described in Chapter 2. This analysis of the incentives in the political marketplace provides a basis for examining medical care policy issues beginning with Chapter 4. The particular policy issues are national health insurance, the reduction of excess hospital capacity, medical care inflation, the regulation of long-term care facilities, and the role of the consumer in health planning. A concluding chapter discusses the implications of these studies and applies the political-economic model in a limited assessment of the potential for government policies supporting a "competitive approach" to medical care reform.

—TRM and JBC

Chapter 1

Policies Toward Medical Care

Expectations and Performance

The early 1960s were prosperous years in the United States by almost any measure. Real incomes rose by 5 to 10 percent annually, the yearly inflation rate hovered between 1 and 2 percent, and unemployment rates reached lows of 3 to 4 percent. Yet, even in the midst of this general prosperity, there seemed to be promises that were not being fulfilled by our market economy. For instance, the jobless rate among blacks was much higher than that of whites, inner-city areas were decaying at an alarming rate, transportation systems and schools in many urban areas seemed inadequate, and substantial segments of the population both in urban and rural areas had much lower living standards than the norm.

The relatively low levels of consumption, among subgroups of the population, of such "basic" commodities as food, housing, clothing, education, and medical care were highlighted by the general prosperity of the times. It seemed clear to many that this disparity was a consequence of a market-oriented economy and that "private enterprise" could not be expected to correct the situation. Therefore, additional government intervention in traditionally private market transactions commonly was viewed as necessary and desirable.

The intellectual case for increased public sector action was based on the developing field of "welfare economics." The theory of welfare economics identifies the necessary and sufficient conditions for a market economy to generate a socially optimal production and distribution of goods and services. However, it also identifies the conditions under which these results may not be forthcoming. The vast potential for "market failure" outlined in this literature apparently provides theoretical justification for government participation in the production as well as the distribution of almost every good or service.

Conditions therefore were advantageous for government expansion of its activities in the private sector, particularly as they related to basic consumer goods and services. A constituency supported such efforts, welfare economics provided some intellectual justification, and a healthy economy provided the means. Therefore, during the middle and late 1960s there was an unprecedented expansion of government support for "social welfare" programs. Federal government spending for cash support programs, in-kind transfers, and other social programs increased from $23 billion in 1960 to $149.6 billion in 1975. These programs increased their federal budget share from 24.9 percent to 49.1 percent in the same period.[1]

Government activity in the market for medical care during this time did not increase as fast as in other areas; nevertheless the expansion was substantial.[2] Total private and public spending for medical care grew from approximately $26 billion in 1960 to almost $120 billion in 1975,[3] or $50 billion in 1960 dollars, after adjusting for increases in medical care prices. Public spending increased from 25 to 42 percent of total spending during the same period. Of the $45.6 billion in public spending for medical care in 1975, about $31 billion were dispersed by the federal government. The Medicare and Medicaid programs accounted for about $28 billion of total government expenditures in 1975, with the remaining $17.6 billion spent on a wide range of other medical care programs.[4]

Some of the programs instituted in the 1960s have since been abandoned or redesigned (for instance, regional medical programs and neighborhood health centers), but others have survived and expanded their scope and budgets (Medicaid).

The medical care programs proposed or adopted in the past fifteen years invariably have taken their aims from one or more familiar criticisms of the performance of the private market: (1) The price of medical care and the proportion of income devoted to its purchase have been increasing rapidly; (2) there is an uneven geographical distribution of medical care resources, with relative scarcity in many inner-city and rural areas; and/or (3) there is disparity in the consumption of medical care between the poor and the upper-income classes.

Expectation and Performance

In the late 1970s, an extensive literature developed that critically evaluated government medical care programs initiated during the 1960s and early 1970s. As this literature reveals, the achievement of program objectives has been disappointing in many respects. To illustrate the nature of these results, some evaluations of government programs in four areas are summarized below.

Controlling Hospital Expansion

The existence of hospital beds is believed by some researchers to induce their utilization. The logic behind this belief, according to O'Donoghue, is that "if the occupancy rate is relatively low there is a decrease in the pressure on physicians to keep patients out of the hospital or get them out of the hospital faster. . . . In contrast, if the occupancy rate is high, then there is an incentive for physicians to treat patients outside the hospital and to move them through the hospital relatively rapidly."[5] If this is correct, then the supply of hospital beds could be limited with little effect on patient health but with considerable cost savings.

On the basis of this possibility, certificate-of-need legislation gave state-designated agencies the power to reject hospital decisions to build, expand, or modernize their physical plants or expend more than some designated amount on new equipment. By 1976 there were certificate-of-need laws in twenty-four states and similar legislation in seven others. Furthermore, the National Health Planning and Resources Development Act (1974) extended the authorization of certificate-of-need programs to all states.

In the early 1970s, when the certificate-of-need concept first became popular, some analysts expressed doubts about its likely operational effectiveness.[6] These doubts centered on the capacity and willingness of regulatory agencies to carry out their mandates and/or the unanticipated effects that might be forthcoming if they did.

Several studies have attempted to assess the impact of certificate-of-need programs.[7] Salkever and Bice found that early certificate-of-need (CON) programs controlled the construction of new beds, but stimulated other types of investment expenditures in hospitals, resulting in little change in expenditure per bed.[8] Presumably this occurs as hospitals shift their expenditures away from building beds and toward the purchase of equipment. Such equipment is demanded by physicians and can be justified on the basis of "medical need." Salkever and Bice point out that tighter regulation is not necessarily called for in these circumstances. The cost of regulating each hospital equipment purchase of any substantial magnitude may well outweigh any potential cost savings.

Hellinger also found no evidence that certificate-of-need legislation lowered hospital investment.[9] Furthermore, he found some support for the theory that "hospitals anticipated the effect of certificate-of-need legislation by increasing investment in the period preceding the enactment of the legislation."[9] Thus they were able to alter their behavior so as to escape the initial impact of the legislation.

Sloan and Steinwald,[10] employing a more sophisticated model and a more comprehensive data set, generally confirmed the findings of Salkever and Bice. They found that hospitals respond to restrictions on bed supply by increasing expenditures in other areas. However, in contrast to Salkever and

Bice, Sloan and Steinwald concluded that this spending occurs for labor, rather than capital, inputs.

Influencing Distribution of Physicians

Physicians are distributed unequally throughout the United States, with relatively few located in rural areas. Numerous studies have offered possible explanations for this maldistribution. Some have argued that a "threshold population" is needed to provide rural physicians with adequate income potential. Others have identified prior exposure to rural areas, the "quality" of rural life, the availability of a hospital, and the opportunity to join a group practice as important factors in physician decisions about where to practice.

A multitude of government programs have emerged to lure physicians to rural areas, most based on the factors cited above. These programs offer scholarships, loan forgiveness, and liability insurance, all of which effectively increase physician incomes. In addition there are rural preceptorships and the National Health Service Corps to acquaint physicians with the rural life and practice.

Eisenberg and Cantwell summarized both the provisions of these programs and the evidence of their effectiveness. They concluded that "programs which have relied on financial incentives have met with less than anticipated successes."[11] For example, loan-forgiveness programs were in operation in seventeen states in 1970. They typically offered tuition loans to medical students who agreed to practice for a predetermined length of time in a "doctor-shortage" area. Either all or a portion of the loan was forgiven upon fulfillment of the practice obligation, or physicians were released from this obligation if their loans were repaid in cash. In an evaluation of these programs, Mason discovered that at least one-third of the loan recipients exercised their "buy-out" options.[12] Lewis et al., in examining eleven loan-forgiveness programs, found that "they have had limited success in locating small numbers of physicians in rural or medically underserved areas for short periods."[13]

Fein concludes that "at current levels they affect few decisions. At higher levels they are likely to be costly, to yield a relatively low return per dollar expended, and to have unfavorable side effects on equity, on the characteristics of medical students, and on the distribution of practicing physicians by income group."[14]

Rural preceptorship programs also have had a questionable impact on the location of physicians in underserved areas. These programs give students the opportunity to practice in a rural area as an alternative to a hospital-based training program. The hope is that students, once exposed to this type of practice setting, will be favorably disposed to practice in a similar location upon completion of their training. After a careful study of these programs, Steinwald and Steinwald (1979) state that "the influence of rural program participation on the practice location decisions of young physicians [was] slight."[15] Furthermore, Fein does not hold out very much hope for the success of such programs in the future: "Unless the more basic phenomena that lead students away from rural (and inner-city) practice are addressed . . . rural preceptorship programs will prove insufficient."[16]

The National Health Service Corps (NHSC) represents yet another attempt to draw physicians into underserved areas. The Corps, established in 1970, places physicians and other personnel in medical-service-shortage areas for two-year periods. Evaluation of the Corps' performance is complicated by the fact that "program objectives [were] broad, ill defined, and have changed rapidly."[17] Much of the existing research has addressed the retention of Corps physicians in rural communities beyond the two-year assignment period. Until 1973 only 2 percent of Corps personnel remained in their assigned areas after completing their service requirements. Subsequently, the percentage remaining increased to 25 percent, however, the actual numbers of participating personnel decreased. Sites with the greatest need for medical services have experienced the most difficulty in retaining physicians.[18]

The success of the Corps in recruiting during its early years seems to have been directly related to the "doctor draft"; that is, the Corps was an alternative to military service. The growth of a scholarship program associated with Corps service has improved the ability of the Corps to recruit in recent years. However, based on the early experience of the Corps, the program's impact on access in areas of shortages appears to have been rather limited.

The National Health Service Corps, loan-forgiveness programs, and rural preceptorships are but three of many initiatives aimed at redistributing medical manpower into shortage areas. The development of new categories of health personnel, increases in medical school capacities, the definition of the "family practice" specialty, and the use of federal funds to construct hospitals in rural areas are efforts that have this goal as one of their justifications. Yet the unsatisfactory level of medical services in rural areas remains one of the more intractable problems of our medical care system.

Financing Medical Care for the Poor

The Medicaid program was authorized under Title XIX of the 1965 Social Security Act amendments. The broad goals of the program were to improve the access of low-income individuals to mainstream medical care and relieve them of the high costs associated with this care. State funds finance Medicaid, matched by federal contributions that vary inversely with state per capita incomes. States are responsible for administering the program and determining eligible clientele within limits defined by federal guidelines.

As Karen Davis has observed, "Medicaid is viewed by many liberals and fiscal conservatives alike as a classical example of the futility of simply 'throwing money at a problem.' "[18] The dissatisfaction with Medicaid stems primarily from its high cost and secondarily from its shortcomings in delivering services to target groups.

Initial cost estimates for the Medicaid program were in the range of $1.5 billion annually but the annual outlay for 1968 was $3.45 billion.[19] In fiscal year 1976, program cost was estimated at $14.2 billion, with $7.8 billion of that sum provided through federal contributions.[20] Medicaid is now the largest single program for the poor in terms of public outlays. This tremendous disparity between anticipated and actual program costs led to a series of amendments to the Social Security Act (1967, 1969, 1972) designed to cut back on mandated benefits, impose cost-sharing on beneficiaries, and monitor the program's hospital utilization.[21] Furthermore, some states have reduced their payments to physicians treating Medicaid patients. While helping to control cost increases somewhat, these steps have limited the ability of the program to achieve its stated goals.

While the direct program costs of Medicaid are great, many would argue that its indirect costs have been equally large. Lewis et al. state that Medicaid (and Medicare) has "contributed markedly to this escalation (in medical care prices) by increasing the demands for health care in the face of a fixed supply of services."[22] These cost increases have been borne by all population groups and have made the purchase of medical care especially difficult for the "near poor" not eligible for Medicaid.

In addition to the high cost of Medicaid, there is substantial variation across states in the consumption of medical services by beneficiaries, with low-income individuals in the South at a relative disadvantage. Furthermore, within states urban whites "receive a disproportionately large share of Medicaid benefits."[23] The program has apparently had little effect on the source of primary care chosen by participants, and therefore has not facilitated their entry into the world of "middle-class medicine."[24]

In a sense, much of the general dissatisfaction with the Medicaid program was precipitated by its success in reaching eligible individuals.[25] Enrollment grew from 5.2 million in FY 1967 to over 23 million in 1976.[26] The increases in program costs arose more from enrollment growth and general inflation than from increases in benefits per recipient. This leads Davis to conclude that "the Medicaid program has had considerable success in meeting its original objectives," but that "the escalating cost of the program has obscured its many achievements."[27] That is, although Medicaid has been reasonably successful, "few anticipated the financial, medical, or political consequences when Medicaid began in 1966."[28] Those dissatisfied with the program generally claim its achievements have not been worth the outlays.

Planning for Medical Care Delivery

Public Law 89-749, known as the Comprehensive Health Planning and Public Service Amendments, was enacted on November 3, 1966. The stated goal of the law was "the highest level of health attainable for every person."[29] New planning organizations at the state and regional levels were to achieve this ambitious end, using five mechanisms:[30]

(1) Grant funds were allotted to state governmental units responsible for planning, the size of these grants depending on population and per capita income. The law required that an advisory council made up primarily of consumers be formed to adivse the state comprehensive planning agency.
(2) Partial subsidies were provided to public organizations for regional, or areawide, health planning. Areawide planning agencies were expected to supplement these funds with money collected from the private sector.
(3) Grants were provided to public organizations, including universities, to train health planners.
(4) Formula grants were made to states for public-health services, with allotments again based on population and per capita income. Matching funds from state governments were required for these grants.
(5) The law also made available grants to public organizations such as universities for "health services development," including sponsorship of innovative health training programs.

As Jacobs and Froh point out, "the social significance of Public Law 89-749 is [the attempt] to impose order and produce change in the health system while avoiding the lack of responsiveness to local needs and the inertia to change inherent in a health system with centralized decision making."[31]

Comprehensive health planning, it is widely assumed, fell far short of achieving its ambitious aims. For example, the act neither defined what was meant by health planning nor described how the planning process was to take place. The CHP agencies had meager authority to bring about changes in American medicine; they were limited to making recommendations about requests which involved federal funding. Local planning agencies were forced to devote large amounts of staff time toward fund raising from the private sector and were only moderately successful in those efforts. Consumer representatives did not coalesce into a strong interest group and so proved largely ineffective. In addition, CHP was hobbled by the mandate to accomplish change without interfering with the existing medical care system. This precluded the introduction of innovative programs that might alter the delivery of medical care. As a result of all these obstacles, O'Connor notes the "great dissatisfaction on the part of many with an ostensibly widespread disparity between the theoretical promise of CHP and its actual performance."[32]

The Movement for Change

The government programs we have mentioned have elements common to many, if not most, government initiatives for change in American medicine during the past ten to fifteen years. The typical policymaking process has these elements. A failure of the existing system to meet some desirable performance goal is noted and publicized. This failure is usually blamed on a particular provider group pursuing its own "selfish" interests rather than the greater "social" interest. Since government is portrayed as representing the "social" interest of its citizens and believed able to bring about change, it appears the logical instrument to implement improvement. A government program subsequently is enacted for the purpose of correcting, compensating for, or counteracting the behavior of the "guilty" party. Unfortunately, the results are disappointing in the sense that the original goal remains unachieved and/or the program contributes to a deterioration of performance in some other area.

As this cycle repeats itself, the obvious question remains: "What should be done now?" This question has provoked a lively debate among medical care practitioners, planners, academics, and policy analysts. The various answers suggested depend a great deal on the lessons one draws from past performance. Although these lessons vary in emphasis, they can be classified generally into four categories. The categories and their implications for public policy are as follows:

(1) *Public policy in the past has not achieved satisfactory results because it has not been comprehensive.* According to this argument, policy efforts that approach the problems of the medical care marketplace in a piecemeal fashion are doomed to failure. The market for the delivery of medical care is simply too complex to be influenced positively by policies that address only a single aspect of behavior at any one time. The private marketplace provides few restraints on provider behavior and offers unlimited opportunities to escape a one-dimensional approach to "correct" it. In the words of David Mechanic, "because of the factors restraining natural adjustments in the medical care marketplace and the complexity of private, professional, and public interests affecting decision making, it is extraordinarily difficult to distribute services more equitably and efficiently without a more forceful public policy than prevails at present."[33] The "more forceful public policy" that is often suggested (although not necessarily by Mechanic) is some variant of a national health service.[34] Under such a plan, government might own the facilities used to deliver medical care, with physicians and other providers of care reimbursed on a salary basis. The delivery of care would be organized according to geography, regional and local governmental bodies performing administrative functions. The federal government presumably would be responsible for general policy and regulation.

(2) *Public policy in the past has not achieved satisfactory results because government administrative agencies are inherently inefficient, resistant to change, and easily dominated by providers.* Advocates of this position often point to the experiences of other industries, such as trucking, railroads, and airlines. The lesson of regulation in these areas seems to be that regulators have subverted the intentions of the original regulatory legislation and served mainly the interests of the regulated firms. Insofar as this holds true for the medical care industry, most public policy efforts would be unsuccessful. More comprehensive public policy would only lead to more comprehensive and disastrous failures because of the enlarged potential gains to providers in manipulating regulators. Not surprisingly, proponents of this view reject the recommendations of "a more vigorous public policy," at least to the extent that they increase direct government control over service delivery. Instead, they would minimize government activity except as it promotes an increased role for the private sector in the health care system, and establishes market conditions that direct provider and consumer behavior in desired channels. They typically approve government policies to provide more information to consumers, subsidize new methods of organizing the delivery of medical care, and increase consumer cost-consciousness in the selection of health benefit options.[35]

(3) *Public policy in the past has not achieved satisfactory results because its goals have been inconsistent or unrealistic.* In this view, public policy has ambitiously sought the simultaneous achievement of cost containment, quality assurance, and financial and geographical access to medical care. Yet a policy directed at containing costs can very well reduce quality or restrict access. Similarly, policies that produce increased geographical access to medical care may well increase costs and reduce quality. The point is that our public sector goals for performance of the medical care system are conflicting. It is impossible to move closer to the attainment of one without sacrificing to some extent the achievement of another. The problem is exacerbated by goals that are set at unreasonably

high levels, regardless of inherent conflicts with other objectives. Eli Ginzberg summarizes these problems as follows:

> First, our national goals are too ambitious. No matter how enthusiastically the American people support enlarged expenditures for health, there is no reason to anticipate that the major current difficulties relating to access, quality control, additional services, and a broadened role for the consumer will be substantially attenuated in the years ahead. We can expect, of course, significant improvements in the health care system. However, serious problems remain in our attempts to realize . . . specific goals. And if cost containment . . . is introduced into the equation, we can expect only failure.[36]

This viewpoint does not necessarily support more or less government intervention. Nor does it speak directly to the proper form of that intervention. Rather, its adherents call for a "pragmatic" view of the ability of a medical care delivery system to achieve its stated public policy objectives under any circumstances. "A call for moderation in the setting of health goals and for realism in the assessment of power and decision," Ginzberg asserts, ". . . does not represent a doctrine of despair and defeat so much as a plea for the role of reason in the search for a better society."[37]

(4) *Public policy in the past has not achieved satisfactory results because insufficient resources have been committed.* This position need not dispute the goals of past policy nor the nature of the efforts undertaken to achieve these goals. Instead the claim is that past programs have been undermined by insufficient funding and/or lack of political support. More funds and an increased commitment at all levels of government are needed, not a new set of policies. O'Conner, in his critical review of comprehensive health planning, takes this position when he claims that "the essential ingredient, if health planning is to be a significant contribution to beneficial change in the future, an ingredient which has been sadly lacking over the last eight years, is real commitment to the planning process. This commitment must be made by the community in

general, by the various levels of government, and—perhaps most importantly—by the providers of medical care."[38]

Conclusion

The lessons drawn from our recent experience with public medical policies are vastly different. Equally, the implications for the development of policies in the future differ sharply depending on the lessons drawn. One can predict that debates over national health insurance, the role of "competition" in the delivery of medical services, and other important issues will be heated and that acceptable compromises will not be easily achieved.

To understand and predict the outcomes of these debates, it is necessary first to understand the structure and incentives of the "political marketplace" for medical care policy proposals. On the "demand" side of this market place stand the advocates of various different public policy strategies. Their "suppliers" are politicians, whose support is necessary for public strategies to become public programs, and government bureaucrats, whose administrative efforts transform legislative intent into government action. The activities of these demanders and suppliers will determine the nature of future public sector policy toward medical care.

In the remainder of this book we present ways to evaluate these activities and we illustrate our approach through several case studies of the political marketplace for government policies toward medical care. The ideas presented in subsequent chapters are, for the most part, not original with us. They have been developed under various labels by political scientists, economists, and sociologists. However, a systematic discussion of their application to the development of government medical care policies has been lacking and could in our view contribute significantly to current policy debates.

NOTES

1. B. Blechman et al., *Setting National Priorities: The 1975 Budget* (Washington, DC: Brookings, 1974).

2. Louise B. Russell and Carol S. Burke, "The Political Economy of Federal Health Programs in the United States: An Historical Review," *International Journal of Health Services* 8 (October 1978): 55-77.

3. John K. Iglehart, "Explosive Rise in Medical Costs Puts Government in Quandry," *National Journal* (September 20, 1975): 1314-1318.

4. Marjorie Smith Mueller and Robert M. Gibson, "National Health Expenditures, Fiscal Year 1975," *Social Security Bulletin* (February 1976): 3-6.

5. Patrick O'Donoghue, *Evidence About the Effects of Health Care Regulation* (Denver: Spectrum Researc, Inc., 1974), p. 60.

6. Clark C. Havighurst, "Controlling Health Care Costs: Strengthening the Private Sector's Hand," *Journal of Health Politics, Policy and Law* 1 (Winter 1977): 471-498.

7. For references to these studies, see Kenneth M. McCaffree and Thomas W. Bice, "The Impact of Capital Expenditure Controls on Health Care Institutions," in Douglas E. Hough and Glen I. Misek, eds., *Socioeconomic Issues of Health 1980* (Chicago: American Medical Association, 1980), pp. 21-38.

8. D. Salkever and T. Bice, "The Impact of Capital Expenditure Controls on Hospital Investment," *Milbank Memorial Fund Quarterly* 54 (Spring 1976): 185.

9. F. Hellinger, "The Effect of Certificate of Need Legislation on Hospital Investment," *Inquiry* 13 (June 1976): 187-193.

10. Frank A. Sloan and Bruce Steinwald, "Effects of Regulation on Hospital Costs and Input Use," *Journal of Law and Economics* 23 (April 1980): 81-110.

11. Barry S. Eisenberg and James R. Cantwell, "Policies to Influence the Spatial Distribution of Physicians: A Conceptual Review of Selected Programs and Emprical Evidence," *Medical Care* 14 (June 1976): 455-468.

12. H. Mason, "Effectiveness of Student Aid Programs Tied to a Service Commitment," *Journal of Medical Education* 46 (1974): 575-583.

13. Charles E. Lewis, Rashi Fein, and David Mechanic, *A Right to Health: The Problem of Access to Primary Medical Care* (New York: John Wiley, 1976), p. 58.

14. Ibid., p. 253.

15. Bruce Steinwald and Carolyn Steinwald, "The Effect of Preceptorship and Rural Training Programs on Physicians' Practice Location Decisions," *Medical Care* 13 (March 1975): 228.

16. Lewis et al., *A Right to Health,* p. 256.

17. Roger A. Rosenblatt and Ira Moscovice, "The National Health Service Corps: Rapid Growth and Uncertain Future," *Milbank Memorial Fund Quarterly/Health and Society* 58 (Spring 1980): 300.

18. Karen Davis, "Medicaid Payments and Utilization of Medical Services by the Poor," *Inquiry* 13 (June 1976): 122.
19. Ibid., p. 123.
20. Iglehart, "Explosive Rise," p. 1326.
21. Ibid.
22. Lewis et al., *A Right to Health,* p. 184.
23. Davis, "Medicaid Payments," p. 132.
24. Theodore R. Marmor, "Welfare Medicine: How Success Can Be a Failure" (review of *Welfare Medicine in America: A Case Study of Medicaid,* by Robert Stevens and Rosemary Steven), *Yale Law Journal* 85 (July 1976): 1149.
25. Ibid.
26. Lewis et al., *A Right to Health,* p. 173.
27. Davis, "Medicaid Payments," p. 126.
28. Marmor, "Welfare Medicine," p. 1149.
29. Arthur R. Jacobs and Richard B. Froh, "Significance of Public Law 89-749: Comprehensive Health Planning," *New England Journal of Medicine* 279 (December 12, 1968): 1314.
30. Ibid., pp. 1314-1318.
31. Ibid., p. 1318.
32. John T. O'Conner, "Comprehensive Health Planning: Dreams and Realities," *Milbank Memorial Fund Quarterly/Health and Society* (Fall 1974): 391.
33. Lewis et al., *A Right to Health,* p. 4; see David Mechanic, "Approaches to Controlling the Costs of Medical Care: Short-Range and Long-Range Alternatives," *New England Journal of Medicine* 298 (February 2, 1978): 249-254.
34. Milton Terris et al., "The Case for a National Health Service," *American Journal of Public Health* 67 (December 1977): 1183-1185.
35. Paul Ellwood, "The Importance of the Market," *Journal of Health Politics, Policy and Law* 2 (Winter 1978): 447-453; Alain C. Enthoven, "Health Care Costs: Why Regulation Fails, Why Competition Works, How to Get There from Here," *National Journal* (May 26, 1979): 885-889; Walter McClure, "On Broadening the Definition of and Removing Regulation Barriers to a Competitive Health Care System," *Journal of Health Politics, Policy and Law* 3 (Fall 1978): 303-327; Clark C. Havighurst, "Controlling Health Care Costs: Strengthening the Private Sector's Hand," *Journal of Health Politics, Policy and Law* 1 (Winter 1977): 471-498.
36. Eli Ginzberg, "Health Services, Power Centers, and Decision-Making Mechanisms," in John H. Knowles, ed., *Doing Better and Feeling Worse: Health in the United States* (New York: Norton), pp. 203-214.
37. Ibid., p. 213.
38. O'Conner, "Comprehensive Health Planning," p. 411.

Chapter 2

The Private Market for Medical Care

In medical care, patterns of production, distribution, and consumption are determined primarily by the private decisions of consumers and providers. Furthermore, "failures" of this private decision process are often cited to support the desirability of government policy initiatives. An understanding of the strengths and weaknesses of a private market for medical care is thus essential to any discussion of the political economy of medical care.

In this chapter, we describe how an unrestricted market process might allocate medical care resources. We present the traditional arguments in favor of this process, but also identify the conditions under which its outcomes, as they pertain to medical care, would not be economically efficient. We conclude that an unfettered private market in medical care based on existing methods of financing, provider organization and service delivery (assuming that one could be established) would not solve all the problems of the medical care system.

The Economic Questions

Every nation must produce answers to certain basic questions regarding the delivery of medical care.

How much medical care should be produced? The answer to this question involves judgments about the worth of medical care relative to other goods or services, such as housing, transportation, food, and clothing.

What types of medical care should be produced? Given the answer to the first question, how should these resources be allocated among the different types of medical care? What proportion should be devoted to preventive care? to hospitals? to diagnosis? to treatment?

How should the available resources be combined to produce medical care? For instance, some types of primary care can be produced by a single physician, a physician's assistant, a combination of a physician and a physician's assistant, or a group of physicians. It can be delivered in a clinic, a mobile vehicle, an office, or a hospital emergency room. It can involve reliance on physician judgment or on the intensive use of diagnostic equipment and laboratory facilities. Many different combinations of labor, equipment, and physical surroundings can be utilized in the delivery of a particular medical service.

Who will receive the limited amount of medical services produced? This, of course, is a very difficult question to answer, involving ethical disagreement of the most profound sort. There may be a consensus on one general principle—the desirability of providing some minimal level of medical care for everyone. Beyond that, however, there is little agreement. Should all income classes and/or geographic areas have access to medical care on an equal basis? How will equality of access be measured? Should all be required to consume medical care of the same quality? As difficult as these *general* issues are to resolve, they become even more complicated in particular cases. The allocation of patients with kidney disease to a limited number of renal dialysis machines can be accomplished relatively smoothly when the capacity of the available machines exceeds patient needs. However, when this situation is reversed, one is confronted with the question, "Who shall live?"[1]

The different methods of answering these four questions vary in the degree to which responsibility resides in some central public authority. At one extreme, one can imagine dictators imposing their own preferences on citizens. All decisions concerning medical care delivery would reflect dictatorial preferences, with no weight given to the preferences of citizens. No consumption or production of medical care would take place except as authorized by the central authority.

In a less extreme case, most decisions would still be made by a central public authority, but would reflect to some degree the preferences of citizens. For example, a democratic national health service can provide centrally determined answers to the basic medical care delivery questions but, unlike under a dictatorship, the administration in power would be forced to defend these decisions electorally.

A pure market response to these questions would take place entirely at the individual level, involving no central direction. Individuals acting as consumers and producers would make private decisions that ultimately would constrain the way in which medical care was produced and distributed. The results of this process would reflect the preferences of consumers and producers as limited by the availability and distribution of resources and dollars. The market model assumes that individuals, when given a choice, will act in a rational manner to further their own best interests. It rejects the imposition of another's preferences (whether determined by a dictator or by the "will of the majority") on any individual. In addition, the sum of all private actions under a pure market approach is assumed to be in the best interests of society as a whole.

The Market Process

In this section we examine the justification for a pure market orientation in the production, distribution, and consumption of medical care. The reader is cautioned that the market described is pure in the sense that no government intervention of any kind is assumed. It is not an accurate description of any of the existing market-oriented systems, all of which are severely restricted by government policies. Nor is it a representation of the "competitive approach" to medical care reform mentioned in

Chapters 1 and 9, since this approach relies to some extent on government to establish and enforce competitive conditions. However, it is useful in isolating the rationale for the historical reliance on market mechanisms to allocate medical care.

Consumers

Consumers are assumed to pursue their personal welfare. They spend their limited amounts of income so as to achieve the greatest total amount of satisfaction. Because each consumer's available income is limited, every consumption decision represents an opportunity lost. A $10 expenditure on a visit to a physician means that $10 less is available to spend on food, clothing, or other consumer goods. Therefore, prices are important to consumption decisions. At low prices, office visits are relatively attractive, since little else must be given up to consume them. On the other hand, a high-priced office visit has a very large "opportunity cost" attached, as measured by other goods and services foregone. Therefore one would expect that a high price would result in a relatively small amount of medical care consumed. Figure 2.1 presents this relationship graphically, with price measured on the vertical axis and quantity on the horizontal axis. The consumer demand curve, labeled D, represents the quantity of medical services a given individual would be willing to purchase at various prices. The quantity individuals desire at a given price and the degree to which individuals respond to changes in price depend on preferences, the price of similar services, and levels of income. For instance, consumers who, when confronted with a common cold, feel that self-treatment is an adequate and relatively cheap substitute for an office visit will purchase fewer visits than consumers with less confidence in home remedies. For the former, a high physician's fee will result in the purchase of very few office visits, other things being equal. In contrast, if an individual is suffering from a broken leg, there are few adequate low-cost substitutes for physician care and a

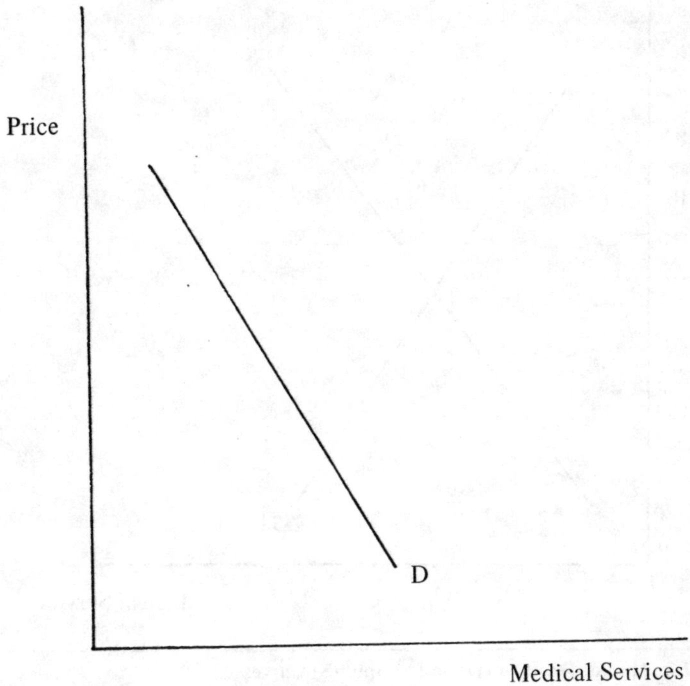

Figure 2.1 Consumer Demand Curve

high price would have little or no effect on the quantity of the physician's services demanded.

Although the demand curve in Figure 2.1 is labeled "medical services" on the horizontal axis for simplicity, there are actually demand curves for every different type of medical service. For expositional purposes they will all be represented for any given individual by the demand curve in Figure 2.1. A "market" demand curve for medical services can be constructed by summing up the quantities demanded at different prices across all individuals (see Figure 2.2).

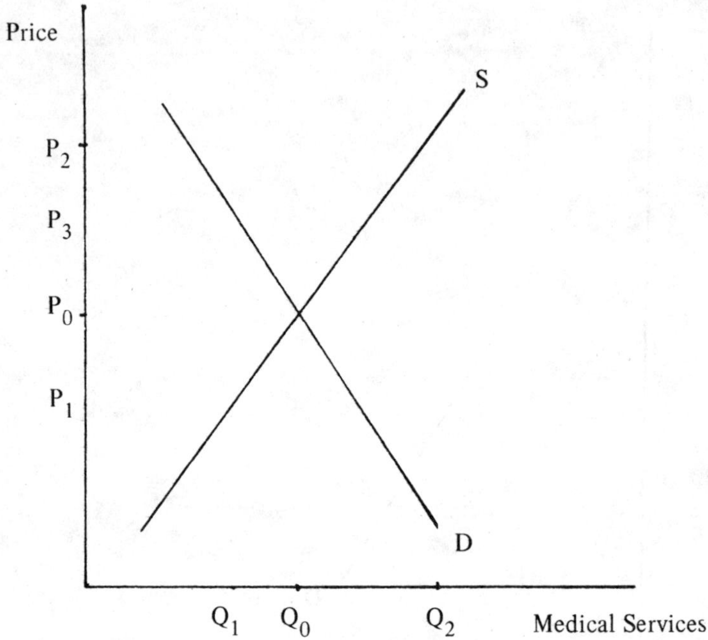

Figure 2.2 Market Demand (D) and Supply (S) Curves

Producers

Producers are assumed to pursue their own economic welfare by achieving the greatest profits possible. For example, physicians, who might be regarded as the primary producers of medical services, hire labor, buy equipment, and rent office space in order to produce services they can profitably sell. The profits of physicians are defined as their revenues minus their costs (including a reasonable physician salary) during a particular time period. Higher prices for medical services can be expected to result in increased production by existing physicians and will also attract more physicians into practice. The market supply curve of medical services therefore will be positively related to prices, as shown in Figure 2.2. The market supply curve depicts the total amounts of medical services physicians are willing to produce at various prices.

Equilibrium

The intersection of the market demand and supply curves in Figure 2.2 (P_0, Q_0) is an equilibrium, since there is no tendency for further change. At price P_1 physicians would be willing to provide fewer medical services than consumers would be willing to purchase. Some consumers, rather than do without, would offer to pay a higher price for medical services. Thus, prices would be bid up until the excess of demand over supply disappeared at (P_0, Q_0). Similarly, any price greater than P_0 (say P_2) would also be unstable. The only price and output for which consumer and producer decisions are consistent is (P_0, Q_0), the market equilibrium price and quantity.

The market equilibrium quantity represents the total amount of medical services produced and consumed, and therefore answers the question, "How much medical care should be produced?" If the market for medical services were broken down into its various components (office visits, heart surgery, physical examinations, and so on), separate market demand and supply curves could hypothetically be drawn for each. The resulting market quantities would determine how much of each type of medical care was produced. Furthermore, the pursuit of profits by producers assures that only the least costly technology will be employed to produce each medical service. Thus, the problem of how resources should be combined is answered automatically in a perfectly functioning market economy, as producers adopt the most efficient production process available. Finally, medical services are distributed to those willing and able to pay the market price for them.

Although the discussion to this point indicates that a market system can answer the basic economic questions in the production and distribution of medical care without central direction, it has provided no normative arguments in favor of the market solution. Why might a society prefer it to other solutions? We now turn to this important issue.

The Market Rationale

The case for private market production and distribution rests on its ability to provide solutions that are economically efficient. To illustrate the concept of "economic efficiency," a term that is quite general in meaning, we again refer to the market demand and supply curves of Figure 2.2. As stated above, the supply curve shows the quantities of medical services that will be produced at various prices. However, it contains some valuable additional information. Physicians will not be willing to produce more medical services at any point such as Q_2 unless the price received (P_2) covers the cost of production and a reasonable personal return for effort expended. Also, it is unlikely in an "ideal" market situation that P_2 could greatly exceed production costs (including a reasonable physician income) for very long, because of competition from other physicians. Thus, the supply curve can be interpreted as a "marginal cost" curve, that is, a curve depicting the costs of producing additional units of output. For the quantity of medical services produced to increase (say from Q_1 to Q_2), resources must be bid away from the production of other goods and services. For instance, to attract more nurses, higher salaries are necessary. The market cost curve slopes upward to indicate that increasing the production of medical services requires sacrificing ever-higher-valued alternative production possibilities.

The demand curve also has an alternate interpretation. The price at any point along the demand curve is the amount per unit that consumers are willing to pay for that particular quantity. The demand curve slopes downward to indicate that consumers value additional units of medical services at a decreasing rate, as measured by their willingness to pay smaller and smaller amounts for additional services. The market demand curve therefore can be viewed as a private marginal benefit curve. It depicts the benefits, as measured by willingness to pay, to private individuals of consuming marginal (or incremental) units of medical services.

Using the idea of private marginal benefits and costs, we can define "economically efficient" production and consumption of medical care as that market solution which equates the benefits of producing the marginal (or incremental) unit of service with its cost. Consider an output of Q_1 (Figure 2.2). At this output, the value placed on the production of an additional unit, as measured by willingness to pay for it (P_3), is greater than the cost of production (P_1). Society as a whole would be better off if some of its resources were reallocated away from the production of other goods and services and toward the production of more medical services. As long as the value individuals place on an additional unit of medical services exceeds the value of the resources used in its production (which is true for all outputs less than Q_0), this action would be desirable. On the other hand, for outputs greater than Q_0 (say Q_2), the costs of production exceed the value placed on the service produced. Society as a whole would benefit by decreased production of medical services and increased production of other goods and services. Only at Q_0 does the value of an additional unit of medical services (as the size of that unit becomes arbitrarily small) equal the value of the resources used in its production. This is the definition of "economic efficiency." The impressive feature of private markets in the ideal is that economic efficiency is attained automatically by allowing consumers and producers to pursue their own interests without hindrance.

Problems with Markets

The economic efficiency of the private market system is dependent on several assumptions about consumer and provider behavior. For instance, since market demand is the sum of individual demands for goods and services, private marginal benefits from consumption of a good are based only on individual valuations of the worth of that good. If individuals do not accurately evaluate the benefits that will result from consumption, then the market demand curve will not reflect accurately the benefits received by society. That is, it will not be representative of the *social* marginal benefits of consuming the good. For instance, if consumption by one individual benefits others, this benefit may not be incorporated in a market demand curve based solely on *private* marginal benefits.

There also are circumstances when market supply curves may not measure the true value of society's resources employed in production. If resources are compensated at other than their true value, or combined using a wasteful technology, then a supply curve based on provider production decisions (private marginal costs) will not reflect correctly the value of the resources needed to produce the output, or the *social* marginal cost of medical services.

Are these circumstances applicable to medical care? Are there reasons to believe that private valuations will not be accurate measures of social benefits and costs in this market? The degree of confidence one places in the outcomes that would be achieved by a purely private market system depends on the answers to these questions.

Private versus Social Benefits

There are many reasons market demand curves may *not* reflect social benefits received from the consumption of medical care. Other authors have addressed this subject in detail.[2] The purpose of the summary is not to provide a comprehensive description of the potential for "market failure" in the delivery of medical care. Nor is it to evaluate the strengths and weaknesses of the arguments relating to market failure. Rather, it is to give the reader an uncritical overview of a few of the more important characteristics of the existing market for medical care that distinguish it from the assumptions of the "ideal" private market, and therefore that might mitigate the case for private markets in medical care based on the promise of economic efficiency.

External Benefits

A classic example of the difference between private and social benefits in the consumption of medical care is found in the area of public health. If individuals suffer from an infectious disease, the consumption of medical services may cure the disease, but this represents only a portion of the benefits from that consumption. People who might otherwise contract the disease also benefit. However, in making purchase decisions the affected parties will usually consider only their own private benefits. Thus, the market demand curve based only on these private benefits could underestimate the marginal *social* benefits of disease treatment. In Figure 2.2 the private marginal benefit curve would lie to the left of the social marginal benefit curve. Reliance on a private market solution in this case could result in the production and consumption of a less than socially optimal amount of medical treatment, where economic efficiency is equated with social optimality.

There are other examples of different private and social benefit valuations that produce similar results. For example, consider individuals who receive satisfaction from seeing others use medical care appropriately. They clearly benefit from that consumption, but this benefit will not be considered in the private purchase decisions of others. Therefore private benefits as captured by the market demand curve will be less than social benefits.

Information

For private markets to be efficient, consumers must evaluate the worth of goods and services accurately. Although all actual market decisions are based to some extent on imperfect knowledge, the "information problem" seems particularly important in the case of medical care, since the nature of medical services makes them difficult for the layperson to evaluate. Most illnesses are not simple to diagnose. Once they are diagnosed, there may be a number of complicated treatments available. It can be quite costly and sometimes impossible for the consumers to obtain the information necessary to make accurate evaluations of all possible outcomes.

As a partial solution to this difficulty, consumers delegate much of their discretionary authority in the purchase of medical care to physicians. Although physicians are clearly in a better position to evaluate the technical appropriateness of a particular medical treatment for the patient, delegating authority to physicians does not necessarily result in economically efficient consumption of medical care from society's point of view. There are two reasons to be pessimistic. First, physicians cannot be expected to know the value their patients place on the alleviation of pain and suffering. This highly subjective valuation varies from person to person. Second, physicians practicing fee-for-service medicine are confronted with conflicting incentives since they earn income in proportion to the number of services provided. Other things being equal, one would expect physicians to demand more services acting as consumer agents than consumers would purchase with full information concerning outcomes and costs.

In summary, the complicated nature of medical services, their typically infrequent purchase, and the use of the physician as a consumer agent can lead to private consumption decisions that do not produce economic efficiency for society. Furthermore, the direction of this discrepancy between market outcomes and economically efficient outcomes is not always predictable.

Private versus Social Costs

There are also reasons that the market supply curve for medical care may not reflect the true social costs of providing services. As in the discussion of private versus social benefits, some of these reasons seem more important than others. But all combine to raise serious questions about the economic efficiency of purely private medical care markets.

Technical Efficiency

It was stated earlier in this chapter that the profit-maximizing incentive would lead all producers to use the least-cost combination of inputs to produce a given unit of medical service. If producers did not follow this rule in providing services, they not only would be sacrificing potential profits but also would risk losing their patients to other producers willing to use the least-cost combination of inputs. However, there are (at least) two circumstances wherein producers may not adopt technologically efficient methods of delivering services.

The first circumstance may arise because the market for medical care is sensitive to geography. A hospital, for instance, cannot produce medical services that are packaged and shipped to some distant point. As a consequence, it draws customers from a limited geographical area. The number of services it provides, and hence its size, are affected in part by the character of the population in its geographical service area. Therefore, a small, rural hospital may combine inputs (to provide a service) in a more costly fashion than a larger facility, since its service population may be too small to permit it to take advantage of potential economics of size. If the price charged for the service is based on the least-cost combination of inputs (as assumed in the description of the market model), the small hospital might not meet its costs. Therefore, in areas that can support only small facilities, prices for some medical services may well exceed the value of the resources required to produce the services in an ideal setting.

Relatively inefficient uses of resources may also occur when the profit motive is absent. If producers are not attempting to maximize their profits and/or if competitors are not pursuing this goal, then their incentives to use inputs efficiently are weaker. Nonprofit producers are common in the delivery of medical services, particularly in the area of inpatient care, where the majority of hospitals in the United States are of the nonprofit variety. The goals of these institutions have received a great deal of attention by researchers.[3] Some studies suggest that they produce services at a higher cost than for-profit hospitals.[4]

When resources are inefficiently used in production, there is a social cost involved. This cost is the value of the service that might have been produced had the unneeded resources been put to their best alternative use. In this respect, the marginal cost of producing medical services is greater than the marginal cost of producing services using least-cost production techniques. This results in both higher prices and less production.

Resource Valuation

Producers of medical services can benefit by actions that make their own labor scarce. For instance, suppose that the demand for the services of nurses at the prevailing wage temporarily exceeded the available supply of nurses. Competition for nurses as resources in the production of medical services would bid up the wages of nurses. In an unrestricted labor market, higher wage levels for nurses would attract additional people to the nursing profession. The market process would solve the "scarcity" of nurses, and wages would reach a new equilibrium level. But if nurses could devise a means to limit this supply response (for instance, by restricting entry into their profession), they could counteract downward market pressure on wages.

Professional certification programs for medical personnel have this restrictive effect but also provide information to consumers about the quality of the services they purchase. The control of the source of supply—the institutions of education for medical personnel—is, however, even more important. Physicians historically have had the greatest success in restricting their numbers by effectively controlling the number of medical schools.

Restricting the supply of a resource necessary for production of medical services theoretically reduces the market equilibrium quantity and raises prices. The unique position of the physician as the consumer's purchasing agent probably modifies any reduction in the number of medical services delivered when physician supply is restricted, but it gives the physician additional leverage on price. Some analysts have argued that physicians can determine prices for their services relatively free of market restraints. They view consumers as largely passive in the purchase of medical services. If this is true, then physicians are able to assign values to their labor that have little relationship to social benefits and costs.

Nonefficiency Criteria

The problems with the private market for medical services make it unlikely that a pure market process will produce an "economically efficient" solution. But suppose that private supply curves did represent social marginal costs and demand curves were identical to social marginal benefits. Might a private market equilibrium solution to the four basic economic questions still be regarded as undesirable? The answer is clearly yes if economic efficiency is not accepted as the single criterion that society uses to judge the desirability of market outcomes.

Increasingly, popular opinion seems to support equality as a moral principle guiding health policy. The proposition on which this principle is based in that ill health, rather than income, is the proper guide for the distribution of medical care. A commonly accepted corollary to this proposition is that those in need should enjoy a "right" or "entitlement" to medical care.[5] In this view, the market solution is rejected because it delivers less than the "needed" amount of medical care to consumers.

A method for measuring need is required if this idea is to be adopted in preference to market allocations of medical services. However, the concept of medical need has proven difficult to operationalize. Therefore, some authors have suggested that, rather than focusing attention on "rights" to medical care, standards should be set at some level that is adequate but less than the "best possible" medical care.[6] This requires reaching an agreement regarding what services are tolerable and affordable in order to define a minimum service package which would be available to all, regardless of income. While adding concreteness to arguments for greater equity in medical care, defining minimum standards also would clearly be a subjective exercise.

Corrective Policies

A purely private market for medical services offers ample potential for less than socially desirable outcomes. This potential is only enhanced when one considers the impact of third-party medical insurance, an important feature of the existing private marketplace. When medical insurance is comprehensive, consumers have little reason to be conscious of prices in the selection of providers or the purchase of services. As a result, it is commonly believed that comprehensive insurance leads to an overconsumption of medical services. It also weakens incentives for providers to be cost-conscious in the delivery of services, since their cost-consciousness is of little consequence to the individual consumer. Therefore, comprehensive third-party insurance reduces the incentives for technical efficiency in the private marketplace.

Given the above discussion, it is not surprising that most government interventions in the private market for medical care have been justified by reference to some variation of "market failure" or to the inability of the market to satisfy the rights of individuals to medical care. For instance, government licensure of personnel, regulation of inputs, and certification of medical facilities all could be viewed as attempts to deal with poor consumer information. Medicaid, which reduces the price of medical care to the poor, addresses concerns for equity and the consumption of medical care by low-income groups. Hospital-rate regulation is justified because of the nonprofit nature of many hospitals and their lack of internal incentives for the efficient use of resources. The list of such examples is extensive; multiple government policies can be found that address each perceived market failure. In subsequent chapters, we provide our own account of the origin of some of these policies and discuss the connection between program origin and probable program effectiveness. We begin by examining the political "market process" that allocates government policies relating to medical care.

NOTES

1. Victor R. Fuchs, *Who Shall Live? Health, Economics, and Social Choice (New York: Basic Books, 1974).*

2. For example, see Kenneth J. Arrow, *"Uncertainty and the Welfare Economics of Medical Care," American Economic Review* 53 (December 1963): 941-973; John T. Dunlop, "Some Facts of the Economics of Health Care Delivery," *Journal of Medical Education* 45 (March 1970): 133-138; Fuchs, *Who Shall Live.;* Herbert Klarman, *The Economics of Health* (New York: Columbia University Press, 1965); Charles E. Lewis, Fein Rashi, and David Mechanic, *A Right to Health: The Problem of Access to Primary Medical Care* (New York: John Wiley, 1976), pp. 5-6, 262-266; Mark V. Pauly, *Medical Care at Public Expense: A Study in Applied Welfare Economics* (New York: Praeger, 1971).

3. For example, see Joseph P. Newhouse, "Toward a Theory of Nonprofit Institutions: An Economics Model of a Hospital," *American Economic Review* 60 (March 1970): 64-74; Mau Lin Lee, "A Conspicuous Production Theory of Hospital Behavior," *Southern Economics Journal* 38 (July 1971): 48-59.

4. Kenneth W. Clarkson, "Some Implications of Property Rights in Hospital Management," *Journal of Law and Economics* 15 (October 1972): 363-376.

Chapter 3

The Political Market for Government Health Policies

In the last chapter the strengths and weaknesses of economic markets in the delivery of medical care were described. The weaknesses of a pure market approach suggest a potentially significant role for government in the production and distribution of medical services. Once a role for collective, as opposed to individual, input into economic decision-making is acknowledged in any society, a mechanism must be established for carrying out this action. In theory, one can imagine all affected parties voluntarily reaching agreement on the proper method for "correcting" each market failure that arises. In practice, this is implausible. As Chapter 2 points out, the number of these failures in just one area—the delivery of medical care—is potentially enormous. Their correction could become a full-time occupation for all involved parties. Therefore, it makes sense to establish by law the taxing and spending power necessary to alter private market incentives and/or outcomes, and to delegate this power to individuals comprising the government. In this chapter, we present one theory of how government performs its role in an economy based primarily on the actions of private decision makers. Although the theory is quite general in its development and implications,[1] we present it in the context of government medical care policymaking.

Defining the Political Marketplace

In the discussion that follows, we describe medical care policies as "political goods" traded in a "political marketplace" with a basic structure similar to that of the private market for medical care, described in Chapter 2. Medical care policies, the commodities of value in the political marketplace, are defined broadly as any government actions that alter, or promise to alter, the production or distribution of medical care by the private sector. Therefore they would include subsidies, restrictions on provider behavior, taxes, restrictions on prices, alternations of consumer purchasing power, and the like.

Politicians "supply" government medical care policies to their constituents who are individual consumers and consumers organized as interest groups. Both constituents and politicians reap benefits or incur costs resulting from the medical care policies adopted. The interaction of politician-suppliers and constituent-demanders through the political process generates the configuration of medical care politicies that exists, at least in statute form, at any point in time. Complicating the simple political marketplace are bureaucrats, who are charged with the implementation of the medical care policies demanded by citizens and supplied by politicians. Therefore, they also play an important role in determination of the medical policies ultimately provided by government. Members of each of these groups—politician-suppliers, constitutent-demanders, and bureaucrats—pursue their own personal objectives in the political marketplace. The nature of these objectives and the relative incentives and abilities of the groups determine the actual configuration of medical care policies.

The Constituent-Demander

When citizens delegate decision-making authority to elected representatives, they assume that their own preferences for collective action will not be satisfied completely. Elected representatives are responsible to a number of constituents, each with different tastes, incomes, and perceptions of the importance of particular issues. Therefore, the politician's decision on any single question is not likely to mirror the precise aims of most constituents. It is the potential of this representative process to confer gains or impose losses that motivates voters and their interest-group agents to participate actively in the political marketplace as demanders of particular public actions.

Government policies, in this view, satisfy consumers in the same manner as private goods and services do. Consumers support those policies that increase their satisfaction and oppose those that diminish it. Therefore, the policies particular consumers desire are influenced by the same considerations that determine consumption in the private market: the price of the policy, the price of other policies, the prices of private goods and services, income, and tastes. On the basis of these considerations, consumers determine which government actions are in their own best interest and then support representatives who promise to deliver the set of policies most closely approximating their policy preferences. If constituent-demanders strongly oppose Medicaid reimbursement for abortions, while strongly supporting subsidies for rural hospitals, they will search for a political candidate sharing these views or attempt to influence candidates to adopt them.

There are many possible means citizens may use in influencing their representatives to adopt specific policy positions. The most common is the ballot box. Votes indicate policy preferences and influence politicians to adopt particular views. One also can attempt to influence representatives through private communication and monetary contributions, or by supporting lobbying efforts, pressure groups, and social movements. Voters have private options available as well. For example, in some instances they can move to jurisdictions providing policies that more closely approximate their ideas and ideals. The actions chosen and the extent to which they are pursued depend on the potential benefits or costs to consumers of the policy change versus the cost of attempting to influence policy. For most voters, any particular change in public policy toward medical care is likely to be of marginal importance. The individual gains or losses such changes generate are unlikely to dominate the attention of the average voter. On the other hand, the costs of attempting to influence particular policies can be quite large. One would therefore expect little effort on the part of most voters to influence their representatives on the majority of medical care policy issues.

In trying to make a rational judgment about particular medical care policies and the desirability of actively pursuing them, constituents are confronted with a lack of information. First, they cannot be certain their representatives will act on policy promises after support has been given. Second, they cannot be sure that a particular policy will deliver the results promised. As Chapter 1 indicated, this is an important problem with respect to medical care policy. As a result, constituent-demanders are faced with very difficult decisions in (1) determining their own preferences for policies and (2) deciding whether or not to promote these policies actively through the political process.

The Politician-Supplier

In the standard characterization of the private marketplace, producers are assumed to be motivated by one thing—profits. Recently, the economic literature concerning the "theory of the firm" has recognized other possible motivations for managers, such as personal salary, perquisites, staff, and sales volume, pursued subject to the maintenance of an acceptable level of profits.

The actual motivations of politicians are a matter of debate. Before developing what we believe to be a "realistic" appraisal of the behavior of politician-suppliers, it is useful to present two extreme views of behavior. The purpose of this discussion is not to create "straw men" for the sake of argument. Instead, these views are presented because they define the end points on a continuum of possible behavioral assumptions pertaining to politicians.

The Public Interest Maximizer

In this view, politicians single-mindedly pursue the public interest in their actions. When a private market failure is identified, they examine the possible remedies and choose the approach that furthers the public interest. There may be problems in defining the public interest in specific cases, but there are no conflicts in its pursuit, once determined.

The Self-Interest Maximizer

Politicians pursue their self-interest, narrowly defined. They consider all policy alternatives in light of their potential contribution to personal income and prestige. Politicians desire to secure and maintain public office not to "do good" for society, but rather to "do good" for themselves.

Both of the above characterizations identify potentially important motivations for the behavior of politicians. However, a more realistic specification of the politician's decision-making process would include elements of both public interest and self-interest. For example, one could think of politicians pursuing the public interest but constrained by the necessity to raise money for political campaigns in order to be elected. This would result in some actions primarily serving the self-interest of politicians. Alternatively, one could envision politicians with self-interest as their primary objective, but constrained by the necessity to protect their electoral image, again in order to maintain or achieve public office. The result would be a mixture of actions, some of which might be designed to serve the public interest and others the politicians' private interests. In this case, observed actions by politician-suppliers would not be consistent with a narrowly construed self-interest or public interest explanation of behavior. Therefore, simple generalizations about the objectives of politicians are not likely to explain the broad range of outcomes observed in the political marketplace.

There is one generalization that does seem reasonable: Politicians can pursue self-interest or public interest only to the extent that they do not jeopardize their prospects for reelection. That is, in general, policies will be supported that appear to gain more votes than they lose. Factors other than electoral gain may at times so conflict with the goal of securing votes that some politicians come to commit "political suicide" in the support of certain issues. For instance, politicians might oppose Medicaid reimbursement for abortion on moral grounds, even when the majority of their constituents support it. For the most part, however, politicians must adopt "popular" positions on policies in order to be elected. Electoral competition among politicians means that politicians will tend to seek and support, or take credit for, policies on issues like medical care that are "vote-generating."

Politicians are constrained in their decisions about specific policies by the knowledge that there exist gainers and losers from any government action. Supporting a policy that favors one voter may discriminate against another. Medicaid lowers the price of medical care for the poor, but must be financed through taxes on the middle and upper classes. Formulating a political strategy that will in total gain more votes than it will lose is difficult because, by the very nature of the political process, preferences are translated quite imperfectly from consumer to politician. The politician-supplier runs the constant risk of misreading consumer preferences, even in this age of the "pollster," and supporting the "wrong" political strategy. The politician's decision is further complicated by the uncertainty about the future effects of different policy options. For instance, those politicians who supported Medicaid as a means of making medical care more accessible to the poor may not have accurately predicted its impact on medical care prices. Even if accurately predicted, difficult value judgments are involved in defining the public interest. More medical care for the poor might mean higher prices and less medical care for the "near poor."

In this atmosphere of uncertainty about consumer preferences, policy outcomes, and the definition of the public interest, politicians have incentives to act as well as react. They can try to alter consumer views to make them compatible with their own political strategies and/or to collect more information about policy options and outcomes. They can be expected to use advertising and other means to shape both consumers' demands for policies and their support for themselves as candidates. This requires financial resources. To acquire these resources, politicians have reason to support some policies not only because of the votes they might deliver directly, but also because of financial support from special interest groups. These resources can, in turn, be used to secure votes through advertising. Therefore, policies supported by politicians need not be favored by the majority. More support may be gained from a minority that strongly favors a particular policy, and backs that support with votes and dollars, than will be lost from a majority of voters who mildly oppose the action.

The need for politicians to collect information about policy effects also enhances the potential influence of well-organized minorities. For instance, in assessing the impact of a hospital cost-containment measure, Congress must rely in part on data supplied by hospitals through their professional associations. It is plausible that such associations will supply timely and sophisticated analyses of the effects of the proposed policy. This gives hospital administrators and owners influence over the formulation of the policy out of proportion to their individual votes.

Special interest groups rarely share the same goals and priorities for government policies, and medical care policy is no exception. The ultimate influence of such groups on policy formation is dependent on their relative skill in pursuing their goals, the resources available to devote to the effort, and the relative importance of the issue to the group. Their role in the political marketplace can be extremely important, but it has no clear counterpart in the private market.

The Bureaucracy

The bureaucracy is that component of the government which in theory is responsible to elected representatives but is not itself subject to approval by voters. Its primary legal function is the administration of the policies enacted by elected representatives. Its role is somewhat analogous to that of the employees in a private firm. Management makes production decisions, but employees must carry out these decisions. Similarly, representatives make general decisions about which policies will be supplied to voters, but leave to the bureaucracy many of the details about how and when general policy decisions are to be translated into concrete actions. In addition, bureaucrats collect, analyze, and transmit information relating to government policies. These functions greatly enhance their position in dealing with politician-suppliers and constituent-demanders, as we discuss below.

The bureaucrat's objectives are as complicated as the politician's. It is clearly an oversimplification to view the bureaucracy purely as an impersonal mechanism for translating legislation into government action. Bureaucrats have personal, job-related objectives that may conflict with legislative intent and lead to less than effective implementation of programs. However, it is equally simplistic to view all bureaucrats as devoid of any notion of the public interest or as "captured" by special interests. It has been argued that the well-being of bureaucrats is intimately related to the well-being of the bureau or agency that employs them.[2] In a milieu of conflicting interest-group demands and often ambiguous legislative directives, it does not seem unreasonable that the majority of bureaucrats could perceive the public interest to be coincidental with the well-being of the bureau. Thus, they will believe, in most cases, that the public interest is served by actions that enhance the prestige, size, and budget of their organization.

These assumptions mean that bureaucrats will not be passive recipients of policy decisions. Rather, they will initiate policy proposals that promote their objectives and lobby for them with elected representatives. Their control over information essential for politicians to make judgments about policy benefits and costs and their ability to distribute this information selectively constitute the bureaucracy's most powerful tools.

Problems with Political Markets

In the previous chapter we identified situations in which the efficient operation of a private medical care marketplace was unlikely to occur. We defined efficient market outcomes as combinations of price and quantity that equalized the social marginal benefit from consumption and the social marginal costs of production. We also discussed equity considerations as they affect the standards for consumption of medical care. In this chapter we have depicted the voter as a demander of government policies affecting the production and consumption of medical care and the politician as thc producer, or supplier, of these policies. The interaction of voters and politicians defines a political marketplace in which policies are exchanged for votes and dollars, similar to the exchange of medical care for dollars in the private market. The common denominator of the policies exchanged is their ability to alter, either directly or indirectly, the outcomes of the hypothetical, purely private market for medical care described in Chapter 2.

Continuing our parallel development of the "political marketplace" in the discussion that follows, we describe the potential for both inefficient and inequitable results to occur when policies are exchanged for votes and financial support.[3] In particular, we identify four areas of concern similar to the problem areas in the private market: external benefits and costs, information, technical efficiency, and equity.

External Benefits and Costs

When individuals pursuing their own private gains do not receive all of the benefits of their actions or incur all of the costs, they are not likely to make efficient decisions from society's point of view. That is, they are likely to take actions for which the costs to society exceed the benefits, or forego actions for which benefits are greater than costs. One can readily identify two situations wherein this is likely to occur in the political process.

First, given the concern of politicians with reelection and the fact that politicians do not incur the costs or reap the benefits of their actions when they are no longer in public office, they are likely to discount heavily benefits realized or costs paid at some distant date. Equally, they are likely to emphasize strongly those benefits and costs that are felt prior to the next election period. If politicians "discount" benefits and costs at a higher rate than is socially desirable, the adoption of inefficient policies will result. Some actions will be taken for which the social marginal costs exceed the benefits because the costs accrue in the future but the benefits are felt in the present. Similarly, actions that should be taken will be foregone when their costs are incurred immediately but their benefits accummulate gradually over a longer period of time.

Second, because of the nature of majority rule, individual voters can benefit from policies for which they do not pay the full cost. If the costs of a policy are spread over the entire community, while the benefits are enjoyed by some subset of the population, "excessive" policies are likely to be demanded by that benefiting subset. If such demanders are successful (and the previous discussion indicates that their efforts have a high probability of success), costs that the gainers themselves can escape will be imposed on others.

Information

In the paragraphs above we noted the difficulty both voters and politicians face in acquiring information about the impacts of policies. It is costly for voters to learn the details of proposed policies and calculate their individual costs and benefits. The dollar value of the impact of most policies on an individual level undoubtedly would be smaller than the costs of acquiring information. When this is true, voters will choose to be "rationally ignorant." The concept of rational voter ignorance has several implications for the efficiency of political markets and seems particularly important in the market for medical care policies.

First, the extent to which ignorance is rational determines to a great degree the influence special interest groups can exert on the formulation of medical care policies. Politicians have incentives to provide policies that concentrate benefits in the hands of special interests in return for their votes and their financial support. Funds collected from special interests can be used for advertising and thereby can be converted indirectly into votes. The political influence of special interests is limited by the opposition their desired policies are likely to provoke. However, to the extent that the costs of the policy are diffused among the electorate and difficult to identify and estimate, the high cost of collecting information will guarantee that most voters remain rationally ignorant about most special-interest-group activities. As a result, politicians will favor policies that concentrate benefits but spread costs, even if these policies are inefficient in the sense that they generate social costs that in the aggregate exceed their benefits.

Because of rational voter ignorance, it is predictable that politicians will favor "hidden" taxes to support policies, since opposition to policies is less when the true distribution of their costs is difficult to estimate. Therefore, it is not surprising that most national health insurance bills rely heavily on "employer contributions" for their financing. The implication is that employers will "share" the costs of NHI with consumers, thus increasing the attractiveness of the policy to the general public. Of course, the employer-worker split, as determined through legislation, greatly underestimates the cost of these NHI proposals to consumers. A portion of the employer's share will be shifted forward to consumers in the form of higher prices for goods and services, while a portion will be shifted backward to workers in the form of lower wages. However, this redistribution of costs would be well hidden, difficult to measure, and accrue over time. Therefore, the actual distribution of the policy costs is of less political importance than the "up-front" costs of the policy. The distribution of benefits and costs as perceived by the constituent-demander probably would not be accurate, and an inefficient policy outcome, from a social perspective, could result.

A second consequence of the costs of acquiring accurate information about medical care policies is the enhancement of the power and influence of the bureaucracy. Bureaucracies will use their access to and control over information to supply information selectively to politicians and the public. The complexity of the incentives in medical care delivery and the "medical mystique" in general aid the bureaucracy in controlling the flow of information. Bureaucrats will use their control over information to emphasize the benefits and underestimate the costs of policies they administer, thus increasing the likelihood that such policies will receive approval. Since cost overruns could precipitate larger bureau budgets, there are some gains from an initial underestimate. (However, there may be long-run political costs to a bureau that consistently overemphasizes policy benefits or underestimates costs.) Also, bureaucrats will tend to favor the introduction of complicated and elaborate policies to correct past policy failures rather than the abandonment of ill-fated policies. The former could increase the size of the bureau, while the latter could reduce it. (Thus bureaucrats can be expected to support the view that past government medical care policy failures resulted from a lack of sufficient monetary or intellectual commitment and were not due to any inherent weakness in the policy itself.) Both factors increase the likelihood that policies will be adopted for which the social costs exceed the social benefits.

In essence, when information about medical care policies and policy outcomes is costly to obtain, policies that do not meet the basic criterion of economic efficiency are more likely to be adopted. Thus, while poor or costly information is often the cause of private market failure in the delivery of medical care, it can have an equally serious impact on the efficient functioning of the political marketplace in the formulation of medical care policies.

Technical Efficiency

The private market is technically inefficient when it fails to produce medical services in a cost-effective manner. The existence of monopoly and the importance of the voluntary, not-for-profit sector were cited as barriers to achieving technical efficiency in the private production of medical services. Public policies that place greater responsibility for medical services in public hands, whether through increased regulation of production techniques or outright ownership control, are only likely to compound this problem. Most simply put, people are not as careful spending the money of others as they are in spending their own money, other things being equal. As a political issue, opposing rising medical care costs has some appeal, but a concerted effort to introduce cost-consciousness in public sector production, regulation, or delivery of *specific* medical services is relatively unattractive. Any increase in cost-effectiveness that might occur through government action would be difficult to identify and to communicate effectively to voters. Furthermore, these cost savings would probably have a very small impact on any one voter, for whom rational ignorance would again be an appropriate posture.

Aside from its political unattractiveness, cost-conscious public sector initiatives run counter to the incentives implicit in public sector agencies. Bureaus are likely to be penalized in the budget process if they are cost-conscious. An agency that exhausts its budget in one year and requests supplemental funds is likely to have its budget raised in succeeding years on the grounds that past funds were not sufficient for the performance of the bureau's tasks. An efficient agency that comes in "under budget" at year's end will probably have allocations cut in subsequent years. Thus, within reasonable limits, bureaus are rewarded for overspending and inefficiency, and penalized for cost-consciousness.

Another limit on the technical efficiency of government is the organizational process within bureaucracies. Large organizations, even when facing the discipline of a private marketplace, change slowly and incrementally. This tendency is likely to be even stronger in a government bureaucracy where performance incentives and measures of success are not easily defined. Thus, any medical care policy that requires new behavior from an existing bureau is unlikely to be implemented effectively without considerable monitoring effort. The problem of "moving" bureaucracies is compounded when more than one agency is involved. Each agency is likely to follow its standard operating procedures and address only its narrow responsibilities, leaving no one concerned with the overall result. All these considerations fall under the heading of "implementation analysis," a topic that is just beginning to receive research attention.[4] However, it seems clear that the technical problems of policy implementation do contribute substantially to inefficient outcomes of the political marketplace.

Equity

While many analysts agree that public sector medical care policies need not lead to increased efficiency in the medical care marketplace, they nevertheless support governmental intervention on equity grounds. The performance of the Medicaid program (see Chapter 1) provides evidence that greater equality in the consumption of medical services can be achieved through government action. However, historically a large number of government actions also have promoted the interests of producers and special interest consumer groups to the detriment of consumers. This should not be surprising given the nature of the political process. Since politicians can use monetary contributions to generate votes, they have incentives to provide policies that reflect the distribution of income as well as direct votes. Thus, removing distribution decisions from the private market to the public sector may (in may programs) not result in a more equitable distribution of services. Political decisions are sensitive to income, especially when the few gain much and the many lose little individually.

Summary

Although most government medical care policies are justified on the basis of private "market failures," they are not formulated and administered in a perfect world. The political marketplace also has obvious potential for performance failure. Politicians and bureaucrats, motivated in part by personal objectives and facing conflicting views of the public interest, can take actions that impose significant external costs on the general public. The lack of low-cost, accurate information concerning medical care policies and their effects also can contribute to inefficient outcomes. Furthermore, the incentives of public sector decision makers are not well aligned with the incentives needed for efficient production. Finally, it is not clear that the political process can dependably bring about increased equity in the distribution of medical services, relative to a private market process where outcomes are constrained by the existing distribution of income. In emphasizing these limits on public sector effectiveness, we are not implying that politicians and bureaucrats are corrupt or incompetent any more than private producers suffer the same shortcomings. Nor are we stating that no government interventions in the medical care market are ever justified. Rather, we are arguing that the incentives in the political process are such that public sector action will not automatically improve private market performance. Although the private market for medical services is imperfect, government policies can also lead to results that are unsatisfactory but are predictable and understandable given the characteristics of the political marketplace. In the next five chapters we apply aspects of these general principles to the analysis of some specific medical care policy issues: medical inflation, national health insurance, reduction of hospital capacity, regulation of long-term care, and decision-making in health planning agencies. The analyses in these chapters highlight the importance of failures in the political marketplace in explaining the design, implementation, and performance of government policies toward medical care.

NOTES

1. See Anthony Downs, *An Economic Theory of Democracy* (New York: Harpet & Row, 1957); Albert Breton, *The Economic Theory of Representative Government* (Chicago: Aldine, 1974); Randall Bartlett, *Economic Foundations of Political Power* (New York: Free Press, 1973); H. R. Bowen, "The Interpretation of Voting in the Allocation of Economic Resources," *Quarterly Journal of Economics* (November 1945): 27-48; Gordon Tullock, *Private Wants and Public Means* (New York: Basic Books, 1970); James M. Buchanan and Gordon Tullock, *The Calculus of Consent* (Ann Arbor: University of Michigan Press, 1962).

2. W. A. Niskanen, *Bureaucracy and Representative Government* (Chicago: Aldine, 1971).

3. References for this discussion include Tullock, *Private Wants;* Bartlett, *Economic Foundations;* James D. Gwartney, *Microeconimics: Private and Public Choice* (New York: Academic Press, 1977); William C. Mitchell, "The Anatomy of Public Failure: A Public Choice Perspective," International Institute for Economic Research Original Paper 13 (Ottawa, IL: Green Hill, 1978); Charles Wolf, Jr., "A Theory of Non-Market Failure: Framework for Implementation Analysis," *Journal of Law and Economics* 22 (April 1979): 107-139.

Chapter 4

The Politics of Medical Care Inflation

The Problem of Inflation in Medical Care

In the past twenty-four years the price of medical services has risen 1.5 times as fast as the Consumer Price Index. The proportion of the gross national product devoted to health care has increased by 71 percent from 4.6 percent to 7.8 percent. Clearly, a continuation of these trends would have serious consequences. Moreover, many economists believe that the "continuing trend towards full or nearly full insurance coverage in the context of a nearly unregulated fee-for-service delivery system is likely to produce continued inflation in medical care."[1]

This chapter discusses the politics of anti-inflation policy in the medical care sector and the determinants of governmental responses to problems known jointly as medical care inflation. We attempt first to clarify the issue by distinguishing between four different concepts commonly used when discussing medical inflation. We then present some of the standard solutions to these problems suggested by economists.

Of necessity, a discussion of the political "market" and the political attributes of the solutions proposed go hand in hand

Authors' Note: *From Theodore R. Marmor, Donald A. Wittman, and Thomas C. Heagy, "The Politics of Medical Inflation,"* Journal of Health Politics, Policy and Law, *Vol. 1, No. 1 (Spring 1976), pp. 69-84. Copyright © by the Department of Health Administration, Duke University. Reprinted by permission. A version of the article reprinted here previously appeared in* Health: A Victim or Cause of Inflation? *ed. M. Zubkoff (New York: Milbank, 1975) as a chapter entitled "Politics, Public Policy, and Medical Inflation."*

with a discussion of inflation. The politics of medical inflation in our view produce persistent expressions of concern about inflation rates, but actions that at worst exacerbate the problem or at best are weak. The most decisive governmental reactions to medical inflation will continue to be reductions of medical care benefits in selected public programs rather than actions to reduce medical inflation generally, until or unless the budget for health is centralized at one governmental level. We find, in general, that a decentralized payment structure reduces the government's interest in effective implementation of anti-inflationary policies.

Clarification of the Problem

Considerable confusion has arisen in the discussion of controlling medical inflation because commentators have discussed at least four different problems under the common rubric of "medical inflation."

(1) Absolute Price Inflation. Absolute price inflation is measured by the Medical Services component of the CPI.[2] According to this index, the annual rate of medical inflation has averaged 4.4 percent over the past twenty-four years.[3] This measure seems clearly inappropriate. What we are concerned with is medical price inflation only to the extent that it exceeds general inflation. If the inflation rates are identical, the problem is one of general inflation, not medical inflation.

(2) Relative Price Inflation. The difference between the annual rate of growth of the Medical Services component of the CPI and the total CPI measures relative price inflation. By this index, the rate of medical inflation has averaged 1.3 percent per year over the past twenty-four years.[4] This may appear small, but represents a total increase of 37 percent in the relative price of medical services over the twenty-four-year period.

(3) Total Real Expenditures Growth Per Capita. Measured by the percentage growth in expenditures per capita on medical services deflated by the total CPI, the annual rate of expenditure growth over two decades has averaged 4.8 per-

cent.[5] This measure is inappropriate for reasons similar to that cited in regard to absolute price inflation: The measure incorporates the general growth of real GNP per capita. Only if the real expenditures on medical services grow at a faster rate than total real income is its growth noteworthy.

(4) Relative Expenditure Growth. The increase of medical expenditures as a percentage of GNP is an appropriate measure. The annual rate of growth has averaged 2.3 percent, from 4.6 percent of GNP to 7.8 percent of GNP, an increase of 71 percent. Relative expenditure growth can be divided into two components, relative price inflation (see 2 above) and relative quantity growth.[6] Over the past twenty-four years, both have been major contributors to relative expenditure growth.

Neither relative price inflation nor relative expenditure growth is a priori bad. People are concerned about relative price growth for at least two reasons. First, it redistributes income to health care providers from everyone else. Second, an increase in medical care's relative price has a disproportionate impact on the poor, who spend a larger part of their income on medical care.[7] On the other hand, the assumption that relative prices are too high implies that prices can be too low. For example, a major part of the growth in the price of hospital services is explained by the increased wages of unskilled workers,[8] formerly among the worst paid workers in the economy. The relative increase in their wages may have been not only justified but insufficient.

People are also concerned about the reduced share of GNP available to other sectors. But as in the case of relative prices, growth in relative expenditures is undesirable only if relative expenditures are excessive on *Pareto optimal* or equity grounds. Critics of relative medical inflation argue that government subsidy, insurance, and other programs promote consumption of more and better-quality medical services than are really needed; that expenditures on medical care bring rapidly diminishing marginal benefit; and that some of the money going to health care could be better used elsewhere ir the economy.[9] It can also be argued, however, that the increase in relative expenditures has been the desirable result of increased access for the poor and better quality generally.

Despite disagreement concerning the optimal level of expenditures, it is clear that if relative expenditures increase at current rates without limit, they will soon become intolerable. For the remainder of this chapter we will accept the argument that relative prices and expenditures in medical care are currently too high and that government action is justified to curtail further medical care inflation.

It is essential to note that limiting relative expenditures requires the simultaneous control of relative prices and relative quantity. However, some proposed policies would reduce relative price at the expense of increasing relative expenditures. If the goal is simply to control relative price, these are appropriate means. But if the goal is to control relative expenditure, they are not. Ultimately, the choice of policy tools will depend on how the medical inflation problem is defined.

The appropriate response to the problem of medical inflation depends on its causes. Some observers have diagnosed six major causes of medical health inflation[10] (whether relative prices, relative expenditures, or high prices):[11] (1) Wealthier societies tend to spend a larger fraction of their resources on medical care; (2) cost-increasing technological developments in medical care in the postwar period, such as kidney machines and open heart surgery, heart surgery, have outweighed cost-decreasing developments, such as antibiotics; (3) doctors and hospitals have monopoly power; (4) the supply of doctors has been artificially limited and substitutes legally limited in scope; (5) greater use of medical insurance has reduced the marginal cost of medical care to the ptients; and (6) the government supplies a substantial subsidy of health care. Only to the extent that health inflation is caused by numbers 3 to 6 is it a "problem" requiring or responsive to government action.

Cures

There are three broad types of responses to the problem so diagnosed. The first is to improve the market, that is, to make the market for medical care resemble efficient markets in other sectors where the interplay of people seeking private gain and paying out-of-pocket for their goods and services disciplines both the consumer and the provider. Such a strategy includes making patients more informed about the market and likewise giving them greater financial stakes in acting on that information. Typically such remedies include the suggestion of patient financial participation through substantial coinsurance and deductibles. This type of remedy is exemplified by Martin Feldstein's major risk insurance proposal, where families would pay up to 10 percent of their income for medical care and anything above that would be paid for by the federal government in a catastrophic health insurance plan.[12] Other critics have argued for HMO expansion as part of the market improvement strategy.[13]

A second answer to this set of problems is to compensate for the poor market structure with public-utility-type regulation.[14] The standard site for such regulation is the states; electrical utilities are an example of such a regulated industry. The standard subjects of such regulation are health care facilities and the price they charge for their services. Many states are establishing commissions that deal with facility supply (Certificate of Need) and, in separate commissions, pricing (primarily for hositals). Massachusetts, Maryland, Connecticut, and other states have set up so-called rate commissions to regulate hospital prices.[15]

The third answer is to replace the economic market with a political market by effectively nationalizing the industry. In this case there is a constraining bilateral relationship between buyers and providers: The buyer is the government and the providers are the industry's constituent parts. The government bargains with the providers on price, supply, and quality, representing diffuse and decentralized consumers unorganized to influence health policy decisions. In effect, the government is dealing with the monopoly power of the providers by creating a monopony for the consumers. The Kennedy-Corman bill (S.3, H.R. 21), for example, provides that the federal government pay for almost all medical care services and regulate the prices of those services by regional health boards in market areas throughout the country.

The Response of Government

For years economists have "supplied" solutions to medical care inflation, yet the government has largely ignored their advice. In some ways, as by granting tax subsidies for medical insurance, it has contributed to medical inflation. Analysis of the political "market" suggests why there is little reason to expect bold government action against medical inflation (relative price or expenditure growth) in the future.

The Theory of Imbalanced Political Interests: Concentrated versus Diffuse Benefits and Costs

The political "market" refers to institutional arrangements —the relationships among organized pressure groups, voters, authoritative governmental agencies, and affected citizens— which determine what governments do. As George Stigler says of governmental *regulation,* the theory of public policy ought to explain "who will receive the benefits and burdens of governmental [action]."[16] Important is the emphasis on the natural imbalance between the interests of mass publics and health care providers on issues like inflation.

An imbalanced political market is simply one where participants have unequal power. This stands in sharp contrast with the egalitarian theory of one person-one vote, implying equal power by all participants. Of the many theories of imbalanced political markets, one is especially applicable to medical care—that of concentrated versus diffuse interests. Those with concentrated interests feel the effects of a policy (whether subsidy or tax, compulsion or prohibition) significantly. Those with diffuse interests have no important stake, great as the aggregate costs or benefits may be. A $1 per capita tax would be a diffuse cost of large aggregate magnitude in the United States as a whole.

The incentives to press claims for concentrated interests are much greater than those for diffuse ones. The prospect of having one's well-being substantially affected creates powerful incentives to act to protect one's interest. An interest marginal to one's well-being—even though large when aggregated over the class of affected parties—provides insufficient incentives to act. This distribution of incentives results, then, in a systematic imbalance of the probabilities of interest representation. It is not the case that the theory of imbalance in the political market explains the outcomes of political struggles by itself. For the outcomes are a product not simply of the representation of interests, but also of other political resources—wealth, information, skill—that fuel the representation of those interests. But the structure of interests does largely determine which groups play a role in the channels of policy action and whose preferences are likely to count most in that process.[17] The theory of imbalanced interests holds that concentrated groups, other things being equal, will be more effective in the political process than diffuse ones.[18]

There are other concepts of imbalanced political markets. One stresses inequality of information among voters. Clearly, vote-maximizing candidates for political office[19] will neglect the interests of the uninformed and cultivate those of the more informed voter.

Obviously, groups differ in wealth as well. Other things being equal, the rich can exert greater influence per capita on election results and political decisions than the poor through donations.

A group with extrapolitical purposes (for example, a labor union), will have greater political capability than a solely political one. The first has already paid its overhead; the second must spend much of its resources on organizational maintenance.

Since the results of most political activity constitute collective goods, the differential ability of various groups in overcoming the collective good problems of political activity creates an unbalanced power differential.[20]

These theories overlap; a cause in one may be an effect in another. For example, a group with concentrated benefits and costs has special incentives to be well informed.

In addition, there is usually a substantial correlation among the characteristics that lead to greater political influence. For example, doctors are better informed (on health regulation issues), wealthier, better organized, and have more concentrated interests than do patients. This obviously makes it difficult to pinpoint the specific effect of their concentrated interests on public policy as opposed to the effect of the other characteristics. This is why the care of welfare mothers is enlightening. On the basis of every criterion of political power except concentrated interest, one would expect them to have virtually no success in the policy arena. The extent to which they have been successful in increasing benefits in the postwar period might be explained by the theory of concentrated interests.[21]

Imbalanced Interests and Inflation

What is the connection between the theory of imbalanced political interests and the response to the problem of relative inflation generally?[22] The theory predicts that government will respond cautiously and ineffectively to relative inflation in any sector. In the past half decade, relative inflation, indeed, double-digit inflation in the early 1970s, has been a serious problem in both construction and medical care, especially since these sectors together form a very large component of GNP. Substantial relative inflation in them preempts other national and individual spending.

Yet, any effective attack on this public "bad" mobilizes the resistance of concentrated interests in the affected industry.[23]

Governmental action to control relative inflation in construction costs would save the average household far less than it would cost construction workers. Control of medical care inflation likewise would cost providers (hospitals, nursing homes, physicians, nurses, and the like) much more than it would benefit patients.

How Does This Apply to Medical Care Inflation?

Who will influence health care most? Doctors, hospital administrators, union officers, and insurance underwriters will have power beyond their numbers; taxpayers in general and patients in particular will be underrepresented. The reason is quite simple. The providers are very knowledgeable and concerned about health care policy, since it is so important to their lives. On the other side, the expected benefits or costs of a health care policy are relatively unimportant to consumers in normal health. Their interests are diffuse, including not only health, but also food, clothing, shelter, education, recreation, and employment. It does not pay the consumer to take strong action. Consumers do have a voice, but it is systematically underrepresented in the political process.

Political leaders, then, have little incentive to follow politically controversial economic advice on how to combat relative medical care inflation.[24] If it is everybody's problem—if the burdens are widely distributed among millions of health care purchasers—political rewards for improvement will be insufficient. A 10 percent decrease in health expenditures—an average of reduction from $400 per capita per year to $360 per year—would reduce the total health bill of the United States by a striking $10 billion. But, while "society" would "save" that much, the efforts to produce such a reduction would mobilize the powerful countervailing efforts of providers.[25] A 10 percent decrease in one's average health bill is of marginal concern to citizens in comparison to the preoccupation of providers with medical care pricing policy. As a result, governments have greater pressure upon them to resist anti-inflationary policy than to act on it.

The main exception is that governments in their buying capacity have a substantial interest in reducing their own program costs. Government departments, acting as if the total government expenditures are relatively inelastic, try to reduce expenditure increases by other departments. There is, therefore, an internal government market which partially serves to put a brake on programmatic expenditure increases. This means that the form of financing is very important. For example, non-health agencies will be less concerned about increased expenditures derived from payroll deductions than about those financed from general taxes. Not surprisingly, providers strongly prefer payroll deductions to financing from general revenues.

Theory suggests that the more any particular level of government pays for medical care, the more it will be concerned about price and expenditure increases. Again, there is some evidence to support the theory. Great Britain, with a centralized public finance payment structure, has a significantly lower inflation rate and level of expenditure than the U.S., Canada, and Sweden, which vary in degree of public support (with Sweden being close to 100 percent government-supported) but share decentralized financing.[26] Tables 4.1 and 4.2 present the changing proportion of resources spent on health care in several Western industrial nations.

Medicare and Medicaid illustrate the complex interplay of the forces we have been discussing. During the period 1966-1970, total government expenditures on both Medicare and Medicaid increased very rapidly; more beneficiaries were using more expensive services more often than planners had foreseen.[27] By the 1970s, the Nixon Administration was trying to hold down these program costs, first under brief price controls with no permanent effect, then merely by reducing Medicare and Medicaid benefits rather than cost inflation as such.[28] In constant dollars Medicare payments per beneficiary stopped growing. Medicaid payments per beneficiary actually declined. Because during the 1970s the number of beneficiaries continued to rise, total real expenditures also increased in both programs, though at a much slower rate.[29]

TABLE 4.1 Total Expenditures for Health Services as a Percentage of the Gross National Product, Seven Counties, Selected Periods, 1961-1969

	WHO Estimates[a]		SSA Estimates[b]	
Country	*Year*	*Percentage of GNP*	*Year*	*Percentage of GNP*
Canada	1961	6.0	1969	7.3
United States	1961-62	5.8	1969	6.8
Sweden	1962	5.4	1969	6.7
Netherlands	1963	4.8	1969	5.9
Federal Republic of Germany	1961	4.5	1969	5.7
France	1963	4.4	1969	5.7
United Kingdom	1961-62	4.2	1969	4.8

Source: The Report of the Health Planning Task Force prepared under the auspices of the Research and Analysis Division of the Ontario Ministry of Health.
a. Brian Abel-Smith, *An International Study of Health Expenditure,* WHO Public Paper No. 32 (Geneva: 1967).
b. Joseph G. Simanis, "Medical Care Expenditures in Seven Countries," *Social Security Bulletin* (March 1973): 39.

TABLE 4.2 Increases in Relative Medical Expenditures, 1961-69

Average annual rate of increase of medical expenditure minus average annual increase for GNP	
France	4.8
Sweden	4.2
Netherlands	4.2
Canada	3.3
Federal Republic of Germany	3.3
United States	2.8
United Kingdom	2.6

Source: Adapted from Table 7, page 31, of Michael H. Cooper, *Rationing Health Care* (New York, John Wiley and Sons, 1975).

The theory of concentrated costs and benefits appears to predict past governmental responses to medical inflation and the impact on Medicare/Medicaid. It has more difficulty in predicting which of the two programs would be affected the most by concern over their program costs. Medicaid payment is more decentralized (federal, state, some cost-sharing by beneficiaries) but is financed by general revenues. Medicare payment is centralized but is financed by a payroll tax. The two factors tend to cancel out. Medicaid may have lost ground not because of its financing, but because the poor are less politically attractive than the old.[30]

Applied to the politics of inflation control in medical care, the theory of concentrated interests suggests that market improvement will be an unlikely strategy. It could work, and the diffuse public would pay lower insurance premiums and lower medical prices than otherwise. But precisely for that reason, the providers would probably mobilize their concentrated interests to defeat or sabotage it. The point about the market improvement proposals is not that they are all conceptually *ineffective,* but that the greater their likely effectiveness, if enacted, the greater the opposition of the concentrated interests and, therefore, the more *politically* unlikely their implementation.

The government—which would have to improve the market—would benefit from an anti-inflationary policy for medical care as fiscal agent for approximately one-quarter of total medical care expenditures.[31] But it would also incur all of the political costs of market improvement. So, the greater the share of costs a single level of government has in the medical care market, the greater its willingness to impose an anti-inflationary policy on medical providers.

Public-utility-type regulation, on the other hand, is politically feasible but questionably effective. The demand for state regulation is partly a gesture toward controlling relative medical care inflation and partly an expression of the belief that direct controls of supply and price can, through state commissions, actually moderate inflation.

Certificate of Need legislation and other supply restrictions will undoubtedly apply only to facility expansion and not to current hospital bed supply. This is protective legislation for present hospitals even if supply restraints will limit total expenditure growth, and supply constraints may even exacerbate relative price inflation.[32]

Rate review—medical care price-setting—as proposed in the United States would be weak because independent of governmental payment in programs like Medicare and Medicaid. This separation of the payer from price regulator is likely in practice to lead to a weak price-setting mechanism. The government agency with the greatest interest in relative prices is clearly the one that pays for medical care services. Again, state regulation of medical care inflation is possible; it just won't work and isn't working in states that are trying it because states pay a relatively small share of our medical expenditures.[33]

The third strategy—restraining inflation by fiscally centralized national health insurance—presents a mixed picture. On the one hand, the concentration of governmental responsibility of health expenditures is, on the basis of our theory, likely to promote serious government interest in restraining inflation. On the other hand, the concentrated provider interests will be (and are) mobilized to resist precisely this feature of proposed national health insurance legislation. Again there is evidence to support our theory: Most current providers resist the notion that health should be financed out of a single budget, whatever their views on the particular form of national health insurance. They point to Great Britain as a "starved" medical care system, where somewhere in excess of 5 percent of GNP is expended on health care despite the fact that it is all publicly funded.[34] Yet, as Rudolph Klein points out, this can be interpreted as an international achievement:[35]

> The British National Health Service is remarkable for one achievement. In most other Western societies, expenditure on health care has been soaring over the past decade at a rate which has provoked an anxious search for ways of limiting the growth. In contrast, the NHS has been conspicuous for its success in containing the rate of increase in spending; in Britain the demand has been for an acceleration in the growth rate.

Health care expenditures in Sweden, Canada, and the United States are more than 8 percent of GNP, despite the range of financing sources from totally public (at various levels) to substantially private.[36] The Kennedy-Corman strategy makes concentrated or diffuse budgeting for health a significant issue.

To summarize, the greater the likely effectiveness of an anti-inflation policy, the less likely is its enactment. The market improvement strategy has some promise of effectiveness, but little likelihood of success. Public regulation at the state level has political appeal, but a much lower probability of effectiveness. Controlling inflation through a single national health insurance program has some chance of effective constraint, but for that reason is likely to mobilize effective opposition.

The greatest chance of controlling relative medical inflation would appear to be through the back door of a national health insurance plan that is not necessarily passed for the purpose of controlling medical inflation and does not have a strong inflation control mechanism built into it, but which increases the effective pressure for controlling medial inflation in the future by increasing the portion of medical expenditures that flow through the federal budget.

For limiting relative expenditure growth (as opposed to price inflation) in the hospital sector, supply control is both effective and politically viable because its costs fall primarily on the prospective newcomers to the industry. Their opposition to supply control is outweighed by the support of established hospitals that want to curtail competition.

Nothing illustrates the futility of most conventional cost-control proposals better than the suggestions made by the September 1974 HEW Summit Conference on medical inflation. Nearly all were in fact inflationary and beneficial mainly to health care providers, who contributed most of the prepared papers.

The Summit Conference on Inflation: Illustrations

The Conference made the following recommendations:

(1) Increase the federal budget for health service programs. (This action will increase the relative expenditures on health and will increase the inflationary pressures in the health care industry. While there may be, depending on the program, some

substitution from the private sector to the public, thereby hurting some health care firms, increased federal activity will for the most part benefit health care providers.)

(2) Keep operating costs as close to parity with increases in the Consumer Price Index as possible. (This is the goal of anti-inflationary policy, but no method of implementing it is contained in this section.)

(3) Restructure reimbursement. For example, reimbursement should be on a total budget rather than a line-item basis. This policy has been tried in some Canadian provinces with limited success.[37]

(4) Shift emphasis to ambulatory and preventive care. (While there may be some shift from the more expensive hospital care, the main effect is to bring more health are onto the "insurance gravy train." A good example of this problem is given by Lave for dental care.[38] If the marginal costs of prevention are less than the benefits, inflation will be reduced; conversely, inflation will be increased if the reverse in true.

(5) Initiate consumer education activities directed toward increasing consumer knowledge regarding what are realistic patient expectations from the health care system. (Inflationary and expenditure impact is insignificant one way or another, but it does create some jobs for health care researchers.)

(6) Provide consumers with information on fees and prices. (It will probably result in a one-time reduction in prices of small magnitude. It should be noted that a footnote to the report mentioned that the providers showed considerable skepticism regarding this approach and suggested that it was, in fact, inflationary—no comment is necessary.)

(7) Change the statutory definition of health maintenance organizations in order to allow for more flexibility in assembling benefit packages tailored to the needs and financial resources of particular population groups. (While this may be desirable, it is not clear what effect this will have on health care inflation. Essentially this law allows HMOs to use the optimal discrimination in pricing—a monopoly ploy to increase revenues and profits.)

(8) Do not allow the quality of health care to become a casualty of zealous efforts to contain costs in the health sector. (Unfortunately, this is the crux of the matter, that increases in quality—more comfortable beds, better-trained nurses, equipment that brings only very marginal increases in success rates—have been responsible for a substantial part of the increases in hospital care costs. *Not* to put a lid on quality improvement is *not* to put a lid on relative expenditure growth. On the assumption that hospital costs have risen because of increases in both quality and quantity demanded, then the desire to reduce relative expenditure increases without having any effects on quality improvement is a desire not to stop relative expenditure growth.)

(9) Monitor the impact of the contribution to inflation in the health care sector. (This is a chance for the self-interested researcher to get in on the "anti-inflation gravy train." The main effect will be to increase trivially the relative amount of expenditures devoted to health care.)

(10) Encourage comprehensive health planning coupled with regulatory power to reduce duplication of facilities via the innovative use of Certificate of Need and rate-setting mechanisms. (This is essentially the hospital supply proposal we have already discussed.)

(11) Increase supply of primary care providers and, in particular, third-party reimbursement for the services of non-physician providers should be encouraged. (Economic theory predicts the first part of the suggestion would work but Canadian experience suggests the opposite.[39]

(12) Reconsider wage and price controls. (It was noted that a wide array of provider groups dissented from this view.)[40]

Conclusion

Economic theory suggests that the economic market will systematically underproduce public goods. This conclusion is often used as a justification for governmental intervention. But the implication of this chapter is that moving from the economic marketplace to the political marketplace does not necessarily solve problems. In the absence of some concentrated interest, the political market is unlikely to adopt a policy simply because it constitutes a public good.[41] The political market (like the economic one) will systematically underproduce public goods (and overproduce public "bads"). The political process is unlikely to right the distributive wrongs of the economic marketplace when a similar set of actors dominates both.[42]

The application of this theory to national health insurance suggests sober estimates of the government's ability to restrain national health care expenditures, which are increasing at the rate of more than $10 billion a year. The experiences of Canada and Sweden suggest that government financing on a large scale alone does not reverse the upward spiral in prices and expenditures. Certainly this has been the case when the government uses an insurance mechanism in which financing is diffusely shared among patients and different units of government. There is evidence that where financing is concentrated and service providers are directly budgeted (rather than reimbursed restrospectively by insurance), expenditures and the rate of medical inflation are lower. This has been the case in Great Britain, with its National Health Service. While one would not expect the United States to legislate a national health service, the experience of Great Britain has important implications for the degree of financing concentration desirable in a future national health insurance program.

NOTES

1. Joseph Newhouse, "Inflation and Health Insurance," in *Health: A Victim or Cause of Inflation,* ed. M. Zubkoff (New York: Milbank Memorial Fund, 1975).

2. Some analysts (including the authors of this chapter) believe that the medical services component of the CPI overstates medical inflation because it does not fully take into account improvements in quality. However, since this assertion (if true) would not affect any of the conclusions of our chapter, we will not consider it further.

3. Bureau of Labor Statistics, *Monthly Labor Review,* various issues.
4. Ibid.
5. U.S. Department of Health, Education, and Welfare, *The Health, Education and Welfare Income Security, Social Services Conference on Inflation Report* (Washington, DC: Government Printing Office, 1974).
6. Relative quantity growth is that growth in medical services as a percentage of GNP that would have occurred in the absence of any change in the relative price level of medical services. It includes both quantity changes (in the strict sense) and quality changes.
7. Karen Davis, "The Impact of Inflation and Unemployment on Health Care of Low Income People," in Zubkoff, *Health.*
8. Lester Lave, "The Effect of Inflation on Providers," in Zubkoff, *Health.*
9. Joseph Newhouse, "Inflation and Health Insurance," in Zubkoff, *Health.*
10. For example, U.S. Department of Health, Education, and Welfare, Social Security Administration, *Community Hospitals: Inflation in the Pre-Medicare Period,* by Karen Davis and Richard Foster, Research Report No. 41 (Washington, DC: Government Printing Office, 1972); Martin Feldstein, "A New Approach to National Health Insurance," *The Public Interest* 23 (Spring 1971); Lave, "The Effect of Inflation"; and Newhouse, "Inflation and Health Insurance."
11. Numbers 2 to 6 cause *high* relative prices (and/or expenditures), not *increasing* relative prices (and/or expenditures). For them to cause relative inflation they must increase in magnitude or effectiveness over time.
12. Feldstein, "A New Approach."
13. Newhouse, "Inflation."
14. Fredric L. Sattler, "Hospital Prospective Rate Setting, Issues and Options," working paper, SSA Interstudy Hospital Prospective Payment Workshop (Minneapolis: *InterStudy,* 1975). For a survey of the extent of state rate review and certificate-of-need agencies see L. Lewin & Associates, *Nationwide Survey of Health Regulation,* NTIS Accession No. 236660-AS (September 1974) and *An Analysis of State and Regional Health Regulation* (February 1974). For analytical commentary on these developments, see L. Lewin, Ann Somers, and Herman Somers, "Issues in the Structure and Administration of State Health Cost Regulation," *Toledo Law Review Symposium* (June 1975).
15. Sattler, "Hospital Prospective Rate Setting."
16. George Stigler, "The Theory of Economic Regulation," *Bell Journal of Economics and Management Science* 2 (Spring 1971).
17. These concepts are taken from the work of Graham Allison, *The Essence of Decision* (Boston: Little, Brown, 1971), especially the discussion of the organizational process model of politics. It further uses teaching materials prepared by Allison on "The Massachusetts Medical School Case," Public Policy Program, Harvard University, 1973.
18. Compare the similar but not identical views of George Stigler, "The Theory of Economic Regulation," and Richard Posner, "Theories of

Economic Regulation," *Bell Journal of Economics and Management Science* 5 (Autumn 1974): 335-358 for further discussion of economic approaches to the study of public policy policies.

19. Donald Wittman, "Political Decision-Making," in *Economics of Public Choice,* eds. Robert D. Leiter and Gerald Serkin (New York: Cyrco Press, 1975), pp. 29-48.

20. A government program to help farmers, to give a specific illustration, helps a particular farmer whether or not he has contributed to lobbying for the passage of the bill. Since the farmer's individual efforts are costly and unlikely to change the outcome, he and all other farmers are likely to abstain from political activity. This is a variant of Prisoner's Dilemma, a game theory problem where individually rational behavior results in collectively irrational behavior for the participants involved.

Which groups will be most successful at overcoming the collective good behavior? Clearly, those groups which are best capable of internalizing the rewards and externalizing the costs, that is, making some of the good private instead of collective. For example, those who do not contribute are beaten up (a private bad to the person), while those who contribute receive a special citation or invitation to a dinner (a private good). The analysis takes on many subtle variations. Different kinds of groups are better at policing themselves for correct behavior (smaller groups versus larger and more physically concentrated groups than diffuse). See Mancur Olson, *The Logic of Collective Action* (Cambridge: Harvard University Press, 1968). A monopolistic firm in an industry is thus capable of exerting great political pressure on behalf of the industry, because, first, it is the industry and, therefore, the good is a private good, and second, it does not have to organize a large number of firms for political action since it is already organized. For an excellent discussion, see William A. Brock and Stephen P. Magee, mimeo (University of Chicago: Center for Mathematical Studies in Business and Economics, 1975), and for an insightful diagramatic exposition, see John Chamberlynn, mimeo (University of Michigan: Institute of Policy Studies, 1975).

21. There are, of course, other explanations for this particular phenomenon, such as the one given by Frances Piven and Richard Cloward, that welfare payments are a technique for "regulating the poor," or interdependent utility functions; that is, other individuals have utility functions that are concerned with the welfare of mothers, *Regulating the Poor: The Functions of Public Welfare* (New York: Random House, 1971).

22. In order to use an essential static model to explain the response of the opolitical system to a dynamic situation (inflation), we shall assume that concentrated interests have not completely exhausted the benefits of concentration and still have marginal influence that is greater than that of the diffuse interests.

There have been several papers written on the relationship of the political process to aggregate inflation and other macroeconomics variables. For example, see Robert Gordon, "The Politics of Inflation," National Bureau of Economic Research Conference on Economic Analysis of Political Behavior, 1975; Bruno Frey, "A Politico-Economic System: A Simulation

Model," *Kyklos* 28 (1974): 227-254; and Gerald Kramer, "Short Run Fluctuation in U.S. Voting Behavior, 1896-1964," *American Political Science Review* 65 (March 1971): 131-143.

23. Sometimes there may be concentrated interests who will fight inflation (for example, the purchasers of intermediate goods). However, these are relatively weak in medical care and construction. Everyone would be for the public good (or against the public bad) if the gainers could bribe the losers; however, the high cost of bargaining across issues effectively prevents this theoretical possibility from taking place.

24. It may be in the interest of the politician to act as an entrepreneur in discovering public goods and offering policies that promote public goods. However, we doubt that it is complete—that all public goods are captured by politicians. For more information concerning entrepreneurialism, see Norman Froehlich, Joe Oppenheimer and Oran Young, *Political Leadership and Collective Goods* (Princeton, NJ: Princeton University Press, 1971).

25. Of course, some providers might benefit from a decrease in expenditures and clearly some customers would benefit from increased health expenditures; but we *believe* that intergroup conflict and variation is greater than the intragroup variation.

26. Odin Anderson, *Health Care: Can There Be Equity? The United States, Sweden and England* (New York: John Wiley, 1975); R. D. Fraser, "Overview: Canadian National Health Insurance," paper presented at the Conference of Canadian Health Economists, Queens University, Ontario, September 1974; and Theodore Marmor et al., "Canadian National Health Insurance: Policy Implications for the United States," *Policy Sciences* (December 1975). Also, in different form, see Spyros Andrepoulos, ed., *National Health Insurance* (New York: John Wiley, 1975).

27. U.S. Department of Health, Education, and Welfare, *Expenditures for Personal Health Services: National Trends and Variations—1953-1970,* by Ronald Andersen et al., DHEW Publication No. (HRA) 74-3105 (Washington, DC: Bureau of Health Services Research and Evaluation, 1973); and U.S. Department of Health, Education, and Welfare, *Health Service Use: National Trends and Variations—1953-1971,* by Ronald Andersen et al., DHEW Publication No. (HSM) 73-3004 (Washington, DC: National Center for Health Services Research and Development, 1972).

28. Robert Stevens and Rosemary Stevens, *Welfare Medicine in America: A Case Study of Medicaid* (New York: Free Press, 1974).

29. Karen Davis, "The Impact of Inflation and Unemployment on Health Care of Low Income People," in Zubkoff, *Health.*

30. Stevens and Stevens. *Welfare Medicine in America.*

31. Social Security Administration, *Background Information on Medical Expenditures, Prices and Costs* (Washington, DC: Office of Research and Statistics, September 1974).

32. Of course, there are models of hospital regulation that could have desirable effects on inflation. If unnecessary beds were excluded from cost reimbursement as one of our referees suggests is possible, both price and expenditure growth *could* be moderated.

33. L. Lewin, Ann Somers, and Herman Somers, "Issues in the Structure and Administration of State Health Cost Regulation."

34. Milton Friedman, "Leonard Woodcock's Free Lunch," *Newsweek,* 21 April 1975.

35. Rudolph Klein, ed., *Social Policy and Public Expenditure 1975: Inflation and Priorities* (London: Centre for Studies in Social Policy, 1975), p. 83.

36. U.S., Department of Health, Education, and Welfare, *Health Service Use: National Trends and Variations—1953-1971;* R. D. Fraser, "Overview: Canadian National Health Insurance"; and Marmor et al., "Canadian National Health Insurance."

37. Andreopoulos, ed., *National Health Insurance* (especially chapters by R. G. Evans, M. LeClair, and T. R. Marmor).

38. Lester Lave, "The Effect of Inflation on Providers," in Zubkoff, *Health.*

39. Robert G. Evans, "Beyond the Medical Marketplace: Expenditure, Utilization, and Pricing of Insured Health Care in Canada," in Andreopoulos, *National Health Insurance.*

40. For a discussion of how the controls worked, see Paul Ginsburg, "The Economic Stabilization Program," in Zubkoff, *Health.*

41. Robert R. Alford, *Health Care Politics: Ideological and Interest Group Barriers to Reform* (Chicago: University of Chicago Press, 1974).

42. The question of the precise comparative advantage of these respective markets has not been systematically studied.

Chapter 5

National Health Insurance

I. National Health Insurance and American Politics

A campaign issue for Theodore Roosevelt on the Bull Moose ticket in 1912, universal national health insurance (NHI), remains controversial.[1] Although substantively about medical care financing, the controversy is best understood in terms of "redistributive" politics[2] since it is characterized by the opposition of large national pressure groups locked into stable coalitions and is markedly ideological in nature, with the political struggle centralized at the federal level and monitored by the national media. As was the case with Social Security, federal aid to education, and Medicare, the conflict over NHI centers on the question of the scope of government involvement in organizing, financing, and redistributing social services.

This conflict has been intense and emotional. For the major participants, the redistribution of income, influence, and status, along with the legitimacy of highly valued political beliefs and symbols, are at stake. On one side there are those whose basic objective always has been to shift medical care

Authors' Note: *From M. Kenneth Bowler, Robert T. Kudrle, and Theodore R. Marmor, with the assistance of Amy Bridges, "The Political Economy of National Health Insurance,"* Journal of Health Politics, Policy and Law, *Vol. 2, No. 1 (Spring 1977), pp. 100-133. Copyright© 1977 by the Department of Health Administration, Duke University. Reprinted by permission.*

The authors gratefully acknowledge useful criticisms and suggestions from workshops at the American Political Science Association, Duke, Vanderbilt, financing from privately controlled institutions to the federal government. A central theme in their argument has been that private financing of medical care has produced intolerable inequities in the distribution of medical services. They have argued that medical services should be prepaid through a national tax system, assuring everyone equal access to needed care and freedom from fearfully expensive medical bills. From their perspective, universal government financed health insurance is the most important missing element in the set of social welfare measures initiated with the Social Security Act's social insurance and public assistance programs.[3]

Historically, large industrial labor unions, the Congress of Industrial Organizations (CIO) and later the United Auto Workers (UAW), have spearheaded the recurrent demands for NHI. More recently, their special aim has been to eliminate health insurance costs, generally the most expensive fringe benefit, from contract negotiations with mangement. They are convinced that a compulsory, tax-financed health program would provide their membership with comprehensive coverage at lower cost to union families. The leadership of the NHI movement also includes a number of prominent individuals who were central figures in the formulation and enactment of the original Social Security Act and every social welfare program since then. For forty years they have been involved in administering federal social insurance and welfare programs and advising presidents and members of Congress on health and welfare matters.[4] The industrial unions and social insurance reform leaders have been bolstered by a loose coalition of

---

Northern Illinois, and the University of Chicago, where versions of this chapter were presented. Walter McClure, Richard Foster, and James Morone were particularly helpful. We also want to thank the following for research assistance, editorial skills, and typing prowess: Susan Urbas, Nancy Lloyd Miller, and Evelyn Friedman. Parts of Sections II, III, and V have appeared elsewhere in different forms: "Rethinking National Health Insurance," The Public Interest *46 (Winter, 1977) and "The Politics of National Health Insurance: Analysis and Prescription,"* Policy Analysis *3 (Winter, 1977). This project was supported in part by grant number HS 00080-12 from the National Center for Health Services Research, HRA, and grant number 2505 from the Robert Wood Johnson Foundation.*

"liberal" church, professional, service, and "consumer" organizations, intermittently united in their support of NHI.

Organizations representing physicians, hospitals, insurance companies, and other segments of the health industry historically have opposed comprehensive government health insurance, regarding it as a serious threat to the discretion they traditionally have had in providing and financing medical services and, consequently, to their economic and professional status. Anti-NHI groups have argued persistently that the market structure of American medicine is responsible for high quality of care. Their major objective has been to prevent federal control over the financing of medical services. In that effort, the health industry pressure groups have had allies from other "conservative" and business-oriented national organizations, ranging from the Chamber of Commerce and the National Association of Manufacturers to the Young Americans for Freedom.

The NHI debate—though the specific proposals have changed over time—still raises familiar ideological charges and countercharges, symbols and slogans portending a more hopeful or fearful future from an expansion of the government's role in medical care.[5] The key symbols have included assurance of greater "equality" and "security" under government-financed NHI, versus threats of "socialized medicine" resulting in reduced freedom of choice, lower-quality medical care, and higher health costs.[6]

The national political party and interest-group alignments associated with these symbols and with the broad issue of the government's role in the economy stablilized early in the NHI debate. Unions and other pro-NHI forces have consistently found support among the national leaders of the Democratic party, and the position of the health industry has been generally supported by Republicans. Thus, the struggle over NHI has helped maintain the bipolar coalitions that have evolved in debates over other redistributive policies.

We are suggesting, then, that understanding the politics of national health insurance requires attention to the values thought to be at stake and to the coalitions which form around these values. In the next section we explain how the stage is set for policy choice by the structure of the current debate. In Section III we present competing national health insurance approaches, and Section IV demonstrates how each is informed by the values of its proponents and by the sometimes implicit understandings of the medical care industry. Section V compares competing proposals as responses to different problems in the health care sector. The final section suggests the likely legislative outcome.

II. National Health Insurance in the 1970s

The leading advocates of national health insurance in the early 1970s were the so-called Committee of One Hundred, chaired initially by Walter Reuther of the United Automobile Workers' Union. They renewed the pattern of treating national health insurance as the answer to the "crisis" in American medicine. Some of the proponents and proposals were familiar, as were the ingredients of the debate. Medical care problems were cited as if no dispute over them were possible. Public choice, the nation was told, consisted of selecting the proper response to the crises in cost, distribution, access, and quality. The debate was structured as if the solutions were reasonable responses to worsening conditions; in fact, the reverse was true. Proponents of national health insurance plans employed descriptions of crises to justify proposals whose central eligibility, administrative, and financing provisions were framed of long-standing political and ideological convictions.

The Rhetoric of Crisis

Claims of a crisis in American medicine have intensified in the last half decade. Specters of breakdown have accompanied nearly all of the recent NHI proposals. Though an effective and often-used technique in mobilizing public opinion, the appeal to crisis impedes the appraisal of competing policy measures and their anticipated effects. The current debate over national health insurance has been no exception.

The crisis rhetoric is bipartisan. The Republican administration, referring to the American medical care system in 1969, warned that "unless action is taken, both administratively and legislatively . . . within the next two to three years, we will have a breakdown in our medical care system with consequences affecting millions of people throughout this country,"[7] Senator Edward Kennedy's book, *In Critical Condition,* captured the views of many politicians about the problems of American patients in the 1970s.[8] In a series of articles, *Fortune* magazine alleged that "American medicine, the pride of the nation for many years, stands . . . on the brink of chaos."[9] Labor leaders have maintained almost ritualistically that "there is little [they] can add in the way of new facts and figures to further prove what is generally accepted: that there is a medical care crisis in America."[10]

In opinion surveys in the early 1970s a large majority of Americans agreed that there was a crisis in health care but did not regard it as their own. Still, they mentioned problems that affected them, such as access to a physician, waiting time, cost, and impersonality.[11] Other polls indicate concern, particularly among physicians, about catastrophic financial consequences of serious or lingering illness. This is understandable in light of the fact that a large proportion of the population, under work-related or Medicare insurance, does not have adequate major medical protection.[12]

Nevertheless, it is not patient concern about access or catastrophe that dominates the crisis conception of American medicine in congressional committees but the problem of medical costs, as expressed in the testimony of government program managers, insurance company executives, and union leaders. Hospitals and physicians are increasingly under attack as the alarm over rising medical care expenditures leads to the question of how efficently and effectively the health industry delivers its services.

Medical Care Problems

This assertion of crisis and the listing of problems have become the standard prologue for national health insurance proposals. The problems are serious, but even taken together it is unclear whether they constitute a generally worsening crisis calling for a particular national health insurance plan. The provisions of the plans, as discussed below, address different concerns; they do not agree on crisis, problem, or solution.

Cost. Consider, for example, the most frequently cited problem: rising medical care costs. That total expenditures for medical care have increased explosively in the past two decades is undeniable.[13] Americans worry most about the prices of particular items (office visits, appendectomies, insurance premiums) or the costs of a severe illness. They fear the consequences of medical inflation in these personal terms, linking rising prices with out-of-pocket costs, and they worry about insurance plans expiring just when it is essential—in the rare financially catastrophic cases.[14]

Governments likewise are more concerned about their costs than about total health expenditures. The public sector has become the largest source of payment for personal medical care, with governments at all levels accounting for 40 percent and the federal government alone approaching 30 percent of total health expenditures. The dramatic growth is particularly evident at the federal level; while the state and local share of personal health expenditures stabilized at around 12 percent between 1966 and 1974, the federal share doubled.[15]

Cost control preoccupies Medicare and Medicaid administrators, and other government departments rightly fear the impact of medical inflation on their programs. Although program expenditures have increased, the real value of Medicaid benefits per capita declined between 1968 and 1974.[16] Therefore, the "cost" problem can be viewed from three perspectives: societal, individual, and governmental.

Associated with rising health prices and public expenditures has been a significant increase in government efforts to regulate the medical industry over the last decade. Examples of recent regulatory actions by the federal government are the establishment of professional standards review organizations (PSROs) and the Health Planning and Resource Development

Act of 1974. In sum, it is at least ten years and $50 billion too late to prevent the intrusion of government into America's private medical care arrangements.

Maldistribution and Fragmentation. American medical care has been attacked as disorganized and badly distributed, losing patients "between the units." There are serious shortages of physicians in rural areas and the inner cities. Increased specialization, in combination with various kinds of group practices, has provoked complaints about the decline of the traditional family doctor.[17]

Recent changes in medical school training programs and the interests of medical school students have encouraged those who advocate greater emphasis on the primary care provided by family practitioners, internists, and pediatricians. For example, between 1968 and 1974, the number of first-year positions filled by primary care training programs nearly doubled, from 4,600 to 8,800. In 1975, 56 percent of the 12,700 graduating medical students entered programs in primary care fields.[18] However, the strong long-term trend toward specialization has reappeared within the primary care fields as young internists increasingly favor subspecialties like hematology, oncology, and endocrinology. This trend is demonstrated by the sharp increase in the number of physicians taking subspecialty examinations by the American Board of Internal Medicine, from 200 in 1970 to 2,000 in 1974.

Quality of Care. The quality of treatment usually comes to public attention through suits for malpractice and accounts of the high cost of malpractice insurance. But instances of medical incompetence may be rarer and cause less social harm than questionable and inefficient medical practices. Drugs are not always prescribed wisely or in moderation; surgery is not always necessary.[19] These poor practices may divert time and money from more cost-effective services such as child immunizations and prenatal checkups.

From criticism of some medical practices it is but one short step to skepticism about all sophisticated health care. This attitude reminds us of iatrogenic disorders and places emphasis on environmental reform, antismoking campaigns, and highway safety programs. From this standpoint, national health insurance is not the appropriate focus; indeed, some view it as a "giant step sideways" that would encourage us to put scarce public resources into traditional and costly medical care at the very time that other ways to improve our health are available.[20]

All of these criticisms—many of which have merit—lend plausibility to the fear of breakdown. However, the litany of critical problems implies more agreement among public critics than, in fact, exists. The proposals for national health insurance pose conflicting standards for assessing American medicine and represent disputes about how to deal with the competing demands for access, quality, and cost control. Even if the problems were given similar weight, there would be little reason to predict that similar national health insurance plans would be offered as solutions.

In fact, despite the popular rhetoric about crisis, there is no generally recognized major problem in medical care *except* high and escalating costs. The various other "problems" are simply defects that any sensible analyst would identify, not conditions uniformly worsening so as to justify predictions of disaster. (This is particularly true about access, where the gap between rich and poor adults has been reduced substantially in the past decade.[21]) Nevertheless, appeals based on the crisis premise are numerous and have supported hopes of rapid decision which the prolonged political struggle over national health insurance has frustrated.

III. Competing NHI Remedies

The most straightforward way to describe national health insurance proposals is to compare their benefits, beneficiaries, financing, and administrative arrangements along simple grids. The Department of Health, Education and Welfare (HEW) regularly publishes such digests of congressional proposals, and public finance experts attach cost estimates and impact projections to them. While valuable for appraising the particular features of various bills, such an approach skirts the political meaning of the strategic combinations that persistently recur.

Three basic types of bills now dominate the public debate over national health insurance. Reflecting fundamentally different ideological orientations, the bills can be usefully distinguished by the scope and degree of centralization of governmental authority over medicine that they propose.

Minimal Intervention Measures

The first group of proposals relies on minimum public control over the medical care industry but reflects the shared assumption among national health insurance contestants that government should redistribute the current costs of illness. The American Medical Association (AMA) has advocated plans of this sort. Its Medicredit proposal, first presented in the early 1970s (Figure 5.1), was designed as a federal tax subsidy of health insurance premiums in hopes of stimulating the purchase of more comprehensive plans. It would have replaced the present tax deduction for medical care expenses with a tax credit to offset in whole or in part the premiums of qualified health insurance plans. The amount of the credit was graduated—the higher the income tax bracket, the lower the tax credit.

According to the Medicredit scheme, the American medical care system would respond to a more broadly distributed capacity to buy its services. From that perspective the answer to financial inaccessability of care was simply to increase consumer purchasing power, particularly among longer-income groups. This approach was directed both at consumers without adequate health insurance and at providers worried about the stability of their financing. Its sanguine view of other medical care problems left many critics preoccupied with its omissions. Nevertheless, the plan itself would have astonished AMA critics a decade ago and generated complaints within the medical profession for its encouragement of more third-party financing.

Program would provide credits against personal income taxes to offset the premium cost of a qualified private health insurance policy providing specified benefits. Employers would be required to provide qualified policies to retain favorable tax treatment.

Benefits	Tax credits of 10% to 100% of the cost of qualified health insurance policy; amount of credit depends on annual tax payments with higher benefits going to those with lower taxable income. Voucher certificates for purchase of insurance issued to those with little or no tax liability. Policies to provide 60 days hospitalization or (substituted on a 2 for 1 basis) skilled nursing facility; physician care; dental care for children; home health services; laboratory and x-ray; ambulance service. Catastrophic coverage of unlimited hospital days and an additional 30 days in a skilled nursing facility.
Population covered	All U.S. residents on a voluntary basis.
Financing	Tax credits from federal general revenues. Employer must provide qualified policies to take full premium cost as a normal business deduction.
Cost sharing	$50 deductible for hospital or skilled nursing facility stay. 20% coinsurance for physician care, home health services, laboratory and x-ray, ambulance, dental care. For catastrophic coverage, a deductible which varies by income. Total coinsurance limited to $100 per family for combined physician-lab-x-ray services; $100 per family for hospital outpatient, home health, and ambulance; and $100 per family for dental care. Medicaid to pay all cost-sharing for cash assistance recipients.
Administration	Private carriers issue policies. State insurance departments certify carriers and qualified policies. DHEW issues voucher certificates. New federal board establishes standards.

Source: U.S. Department of Health, Education and Welfare, Office of Research and Statistics, *National Health Insurance Proposals: Provisions of Bills Introduced in the 93rd Congress as of July 1974,* by Saul Waldman (Washington, DC: Government Printing Office, 1974).

Figure 5.1 AMA "Medicredit" Plan (Fulton-Broyhill-Hartice Bill)

Also within this class are proposals to provide insurance protection against financially catastrophic expenses. Other governmental programs and private health insurance would cope with the rest of the medical care industry's problems.[22] The catastrophic portion of the Long-Ribicoff bill covers hospital stays beyond 60 days and annual medical expenditures of more than $2,000 (Figure 5.2). The major risk insurance proposal (MRI) by Martin Feldstein would protect against disaster while requiring direct patient payment for most

	Catastrophic Insurance Plan	*Medical Assistance Plan*
Benefits	Hospital inpatient *after* first 60 days, 100 days of skilled nursing facility care for persons who received catastrophic hospital benefits. Physician services, lab and x-ray, home health services. Medical supplies and ambulance services except Medicare limit of $250/year for outpatient psychiatrists' services in a year retained.	Hospital inpatient care (60 days). Skilled nursing facility care, intermediate care facility physicians' services, lab and x-ray, home health services. Full cost of benefits under catastrophic plan for recipients not covered by catastrophic insurance and cost-sharing for recipients who do have catastrophic insurance.
Population Covered	Persons insured or receiving benefits under Social Security.	Low-income individuals and families regardless of age or employment status, with aid to families who have incurred heavy medical expenses relative to income.
Financing	Special tax on wages and self-employment income subject to Social Security tax. Rate initially 0.3% to rise to 0.4%.	State and federal general revenues.
Cost-sharing	Coverage begins only when expenses reach specified catastrophic proportions (after first 60 days of hospitalization with unlimited further days covered and $21 day copayment; skilled nursing facilities for those who have received catastrophic hospital benefits, with $10.50/day copayment). Total coinsurance limited to $1000 annually per person; $2000 medical deductible.	$5 copayment for first 10 visits to a physician per family.
Administration	Through the Medicare program with private carriers handling claims.	

Sources: U.S. DHEW, *National Health Insurance Proposals,* pp. 22, 202-213. John Holahan, *Financing Health Care for the Poor* (Lexington, MA: D.C. Heath, 1975).

Figure 5.2 Long-Ribicoff-Wagonner, Catastrophic Protection: A Two-Part Program Consisting of (1) a Catastrophic Illness Plan for the General Population and (2) Federal Medical Assistance for the Poor and Medically Indigent.

medical expenses. Continued patient responsibility for these expenses is aimed at reducing the rate of medical inflation by making patients (and doctors) more cost-conscious. Feldstein's MRI is a comprehensive universal health insurance policy

Population Covered	All U.S. residents without regard to whether they have contributed to the program through taxes.
Benefits	Hospital care, limited for psychiatric inpatient care to 45 consecutive days per spell of illness and 120 days of care in a skilled nursing facility. Physicians (comprehensive including checkups, immunization, well-baby and family planning services; psychiatric is limited to 20 visits per spell of illness but unlimited if furnished by HMO hospital OPD or mental health clinic). Dentists for children under 15 and eventually for entire population. Home health services. Other health professionals. Laboratory and x-ray. Medical supplies and ambulance services. Optometrists and eyeglasses. Prescription drugs for chronic and other specified illness.
Financing	Tax on payroll (1.0%), unearned income (1.0%), self-employed (2.5%), with employers paying 3.5% tax. Income subject to tax is the 1st $15,000/year for individuals, the total payroll for employers (state and local governments do not pay employer tax). Federal revenue equal to the total receipts from taxes.
Cost-sharing	No deductibles or coinsurance.
Administration	Federal government, by a special board in DHEW with regional and local offices to operate program.

Source: U.S. DHEW, *National Health Insurance Proposals, pp. 14, 145-155. Holahan, Financing Health Care for the Poor, pp. 84-86.*

Figure 5.3 Kennedy-Corman Bill: A Universal Health Insurance Program Administered by DHEW, Financed by Federal General Revenues and Payroll Taxes. Broad Benefits with No Cost-Sharing and Few Limitations. Would Establish a National Health Budget Under Which Funds Would Be Allocated to Regions and Localities.

with a very high deductible—it would pay only those medical bills that exceed 10 percent of income.[23] Former Senator Brock's bill, administered through the IRS as a tax-credit scheme for large medical expense, was quite similar.[24] The use of a deductible that is high in relation to average yearly medical expenditures seeks to combat medical inflation with consumer and physician restraint. Yet even when the deductibles are income-related, they raise concerns about financial barriers to care.

Major Government Action

In contrast to this first group of proposals are those which call for major intervention on the part of the federal government. The most ambitious is the Kennedy-Corman bill (Figure 5.3), which proposes a government monopoly of health insurance. To insure that "money would no longer be a consideration for a patient seeking any health service," the Kennedy-Corman plan would establish a program with universal eligibility and unusually broad coverage of service, financed jointly by payroll taxes and general revenues. There would be no cost-sharing by patients so that care under the plan would be "free" at the point of service. Further provisions of the bill address problems of cost escalation (by limiting the total budget for medical care), distribution (by creating incentives for comprehensive health service organizations and for health personnel in underserved areas), and quality (by policing the standard of care).

Mixed Strategies

The third and final group of proposals includes a mixture of strategies that call for increased government regulation and partial federal subsidy of the present medical care system. The leading proposal of this sort is the Ford Administration's Comprehensive Health Insurance Plan (CHIP; Figure 5.4). It combines efforts to expand insurance through mandating employer offerings, to rationalize Medicaid by requiring larger patient financial contributions as the incomes of welfare families rise, and to control costs by state regulation and the encouragement of prepaid group practices, now widely known as health maintenance organizations (HMOs).

The mandated employer plans are a way of insuring vast numbers of families for health expenses with a minimum impact on the federal budget. Employers under CHIP would, for example, be required to offer policies with broad benefits and to pay three-quarters of the premium. The employee would pay one-quarter of the premium and be responsible for substantial cost-sharing at the time of use. More modest payment scales would obtain for families in lower-income categories. While less expensive to government than some other plans (a fact central to their political appeal), mixed strategies do not lower total health care costs unless they result in lower prices

Benefits	Hospitalization Physician Services Laboratory x-ray Prescription drugs and medical supplies Home health visits (100/year) Posthospital extended care (100 days/year) Well child care to age 6; eye, ear and dental care to age 13 Family planning and maternity care Hospitalization (inpatient mental health; 30 full or 60 partial) Physician services (outpatient mental health: 30 visits to community center, 10 to private practitioner]1[)		
	Employee Plan	Assisted Plan	Plan for aged
Population covered	Full-time employees.	Low-income families, employed or unemployed. Families and employment groups who are high medical risks. All others who wish to enroll on payment of premiums.	Aged persons insured under Social Security.
Financing	Employer-employee premium (employer paying 75%).	Federal and state revenues and premiums from enrollees according to family income groups.	Payroll tax and premium payments by the age (with federal and state financing of premiums for low-income aged).
Cost sharing	Deductible of $150/person, coinsurance 25%, total cost-sharing limited to $1500/year per family.	Maximum provisions as in employee plan but reduced according to individual or family income.	Deductible $100/person, coinsurance 20%. Total cost-sharig limited to $750/person/year. Reduced cost-sharing for lower-income aged.
Administration	Insurance through private carriers super vised by states under federal regulations.	Administered by states using private intermediaries, under federal regulations.	Administered by federal government.

Sources: T. R. Marmor, "The Comprehensive Health Insurance Plan of 1974," *Challenge* (December 1974). U.S. DHEW, *National Health Insurance Proposals,* pp. 4, 25-48, Holahan, *Financing Health Care for the Poor,* pp. 77-83.

Figure 5.4 CHIP-Ford Administration Plan: A Three-Part Voluntary Program Which Would Include (1) a Plan Requiring Employees to Provide Private Insurance for Employees, (2) an Assisted Plan for Low-Income and High Medical Risk Families and Individuals, and (3) an Improved Federal Medicare Program for the Aged.

	NHI	*Medicare, regular*	*Medicare, long-term*
Benefits	Comprehensive, as in CHIP.		Extensive provisions for home and institutional care services.
Population covered	Persons insured or eligible for Social Security, working full-time or AFDC or SSI.	Aged and disabled, as under present Medicare programs.	
Financing	Payroll tax (3% for employers, 1% for employees), self-employment and unearned income (2.5%) and AFDC and SSI payments. Income up to $20,000 taxable.	Continuation of same financing provisions.	Enrolled pay $6 monthly premium. Balance from federal and state revenues (90% and 10% respectively).
Cost-sharing	Deductible. $150 person. Coinsurance, $25. Total cost-sharing limited to $1000 per family but eliminated for low-income families. No cost-sharing for preventive care.	Same as present Medicare program but eliminated or reduced for low-income families.	No cost-sharing, except Social Security or SSI benefits reduced for persons receiving institutional services.
Administration	Administered by independent SSA with insurance carriers processing claims.		New community centers provide or arrange for services under state and SSA supervision.

Sources: U.S., DHEW, National Insurance Proposals, pp. 16, 161. Holahan, *Financing Health Care for the Poor,* pp. 86-90.

Figure 5.5 Kennedy-Mills Bill: A Two-Part Program Consisting of (1) a National Health Insurance Plan for the General Population and (2) a Revised Medicare Plan for Aged and Disabled Including a Long-Term Care Benefit.

or less care. Proponents of mixed strategies argue that continuing patient responsibility for some costs will dampen medical inflation and cut back unneeded practices, yet collective bargaining agreements supplementing the federal plan probably would result. In this case, patient responsibility for costs would be distributed very differently from the way they would under the formal provisions of the mixed plans.

Very similar to the CHIP bill is the 1974 proposal of Senator Kennedy and Representative Wilbur Mills (Figure 5.5). In the fiscally constrained bargaining of 1974 their scheme represented a more politically acceptable version of Kennedy-Corman. The Kennedy-Mills proposal is similar to CHIP in benefits and out-of-pocket payments. The proposals differ most sharply in the sources of financing. Kennedy-Mills would be run by the Social Security Administration (as Medicare is), using the insurance industry as fiscal intermediary. A 4 percent payroll tax (up to $20,000) would finance the program, with the employer nominally paying 3 percent and the employee not more than 1 percent.[25] The estimated *federal* cost of Kennedy-Mills at $77 billion vastly exceeds that of the CHIP plan at $43 billion, though both are lower than the estimated (1974 by the Secretary of HEW) $103 billion federal cost of Kennedy-Corman.

There are differences between Kennedy-Mills and CHIP regarding who pays. Most economists agree that much of compulsory premia and payroll taxes are shifted to employees regardless of who is nominally responsible. Each employee under CHIP gets charged an equal amount (the premium), while under the Kennedy-Mills the burden is in proportion to income, and explicit cost-sharing is also more generous to the poor.

The political debate over CHIP and Kennedy-Mills emphasized their financial and administrative differences and subordinated their benefit similarities. Partisan rhetoric makes comparison of proposals difficult. The proponents of each plan are apt to claim more for their bills than is possibly justified. National health insurance cannot solve all the shortcomings of the health industry; the problems not only are complicated; they sometimes are in conflict. One may not agree with AMA proposals, but the organization has recognized that improving "any system of medical care depends basically on balancing three strong and competing dynamics: the desire to make medical care availble to all, the desire to control cost, and the desire for high quality care."[26] The competition among these goals is such that serving any two of them works against the third:

> When you link the quest for ready and universal access with a desire to maintain quality of care . . . that combination of factors works against cost controls. . . . If you link quality with vigorous efforts to control costs, then there has to be pressure on access.[27]

IV. Different Premises, Different National Health Insurance Proposals: An Illustration

Ideological wrangling over national health insurance stems not only from differing interests and priorities, but from differing *premises* about the nature of medical services. A comparison of Martin Feldstein's proposals for NHI with the criteria offered by *Consumer Reports*[28] illustrates these important differences. Their analyses are of more than illustrative value: of those presentations not launched directly from Congress or the Executive, they will probably be among the most influential evaluations of our present situation and measures to improve it.

Both discussions present well-defined sets of goals for public policy on health insurance. These are summarized in Table 5.1. The first two goals of both sets relate to how the medical system should confront the consumer in need of care, and the discussions of the two points cover some of the same ground. Both reject piecemeal reform schemes that provide different levels of medical care to the rich and the poor. Both recognize the present problems of inadequate insurance for the middle class, and the unemployed. Both consider cost-sharing arrangements and here the differences in approach are striking.

As noted earlier, Feldstein's plan in its simpliest formulation would pay for all of a very braod range of medical expenditures beyond a large deductible. This expenditure limit would be geared to family income with perhaps 10 percent of annual income at risk. Government-guaranteed credit would provide cash on hand to cover expenditures beyond the limit.

TABLE 5.1 Essential Health Insurance Features

Feldstein	Consumer's Union
An acceptable plan should:	
1. prevent deprivation of care because of inability to pay 2. prevent financial hardship 3. keep costs down 4. avoid a large tax increase 5. be easily administered 6. be generally acceptable	1. Everyone's health care needs should be covered, and the entire population should be included (universal, mandatory, and unitary). 2. There should be no connection between a patient's income and the extent or quality of health care dispensed. 3. The plan should be financed progressively and in a manner open to public scrutiny. 4. The program should provide incentives for efficiency, control over cost over quality, and encourage innovation. 5. Administrators should be accountable to the public and consumers should have voice in administration.

Source: Martin Feldstein, "A New Approach."

A variant that Feldstein favors is to have a lower deductible, perhaps 5 percent of family income, followed by 50 percent co-insurance over another 10 percent of income. The advantage of this more complex scheme is to keep persons partly financially responsible even for high medical expenditures. From Feldstein's point of view, this is crucial for his research suggests that the greatest impetus to rising costs is third-party payment, which fails to encourage either doctors or patients to consider costs.[29]

While Feldstein regards cost-sharing as the most important instrument for improving the entire system, Consumer's Union (CU) regards the practice with suspicion. CU questions whether, rather than increasing cost-consciousness in the delivery of medical services, cost-sharing would simply reduce initial demand by those needing medical attention. As a consequence, they argue that if tried for the general population, cost-sharing should not apply to persons below a certain income, and that preventive care should be provided for everyone. Furthermore, if out-of-pocket payments can be shown "to deter persons from seeking needed care," they should be jettisoned.

CU's third criterion is really twofold: progressive financing and openness to public scrutiny. On the issue of progressive financing, the Feldstein plan (financed through general federal revenues with a proportional deductible and coinsurance) would come off well, and the Kennedy-Corman bill also is acceptable. Kennedy-Mills and the CHIP plan do less well. The openness to public scrutiny standard appears to be aimed mainly at the AMA plan, with its reliance on largely unsupervised tax credits.

CU's concern about incentives for efficiency, innovation, and quality contrasts sharply with Feldstein's approach. Feldstein implies that medicine is a "technostructure" or an industry dominated by persons fascinated by technological innovation.[30] However, for most of the patient population, the increased sophistication of facilities and treatment have contributed relatively little to increased well-being. Much of it, he argues, would never have been supplied were the patient responsible for most medical expenses. Cost-conscious patients and doctors would cut back on these expensive procedures, and move toward new modes of organization such as HMOs.

CU's skepticism about cost-sharing is reflected in its attention to other mechanisms to control costs. It recommends direct controls, including negotiated budgets for institutions and negotiated fee schedules for practitioners; unfortunately, little is said about the criteria by which these schedules should be determined. CU recommends explicit incentives for the introduction of organizational innovations like HMOs, and endorses peer review of medical practice. The CU plan is neither simple nor cheap to administer (which CU openly laments), and, therefore, the best that can be hoped for is high accountability; the Feldstein plan is cheap because there is virtually no administrative discretion and because only a minor fraction of total medical payment transactions would need to be handled through third parties.

Another element of irrationality (actually extreme risk aversion) could vitiate the cost-control mechanisms of MRI. Feldstein assumes that the several-hundred-dollar difference for a typical consumer between the expected payment in any one year and the maximum payment under his scheme will not result in the purchase of additional insurance by a typical consumer. Only those families with a high expected expenditure will buy supplementary insurance; the premiums will rise and this will further discourage insurance by most potential purchasers. Unfortunately, as Feldstein admits, it is possible that a very large percentage of people will buy additional insurance, despite his proposed elimination of all tax advantages for such purchases.[31]

Feldstein's proposal and CU's discussion differ profoundly in their basic approach, and the difference turns upon the nature of medical care itself. As Rashi Fein has observed, "health is different";[32] virtually every major group and analyst is willing to admit that health care is not just another product (a view as old as the Hippocratic oath), yet analysts appear to take two very different approaches to the special character of medical care. Health care is different for Feldstein because it is *fundamental.* Indeed, he justifies public attention to it because of its similarity to food and shelter. For CU health care is, of course, fundamental, but for the typical consumer it is *incomprehensible* as well; the nature of need and of proper treatment is so beyond the capacities of consumer evaluation as to set it in a category apart from food and shelter.

Attitudes toward consumers are difficult to overestimate in contrasting the two positions. Feldstein's trust in the consumer's informed rationality is the basis of his analysis. Given the proper incentives, the doctor acts as a patient's adviser, accurately presenting the medical alternatives available. The increased "early" dollar payment is not meant solely to make the doctor careful out of a sense of responsibility for his patient, but to encourage increased comparative shopping by the consumer. If the doctor's fee is too high or his advice too expensive, another consultant can be found.

For CU the notion of rational consumer choice in medicine is largely illusory. This explains CU's rejection of cost-sharing for the poor and their insistence on free preventive medicine (a possibility considered by Feldstein). They fear that if the consumer faces the real cost of alternatives, he or she may very well make the *wrong* choice. To call it wrong indicates that the individual consumer's judgment is not to be trusted. Collectively, of course, consumers have a role implied by CU's insistence on public scrutiny.

V. Competing Problems and Competing Remedies

The preceding discussion stressed the issue of consumer payment to illustrate fundamentally different approaches to our present problems. We now return to the original concerns about cost, distribution, and quality of care, and use them to examine the health insurance proposals actively considered in the mid-1970s.

Cost

What will any of the proposals do about the rate of inflation in medical care prices? To what extent does increased spending reflect citizen preferences? While rising costs may be partly a reflection of consumer preferences and increasing wealth and quality of care, there is a widely held suspicion that medical care practitioners are simply delivering more expensive care than people would choose if they faced the bill, and more care than can be medically justified. The AMA proposal for more insurance simply would reinforce these practices by putting more money into the medical care market.

Some stress that we an clamp down on medical inflation only through complete federal financing. The experiences of Canada and Sweden suggest that governmental financing of the bulk of medical care services will not in itself reverse tendencies to medical inflation.[33] There is evidence, however, that where financing is concentrated at one governmental level *and* service providers are directly budgeted (rather than reimbursed by insurance), expenditures and their rates of increase are lower. With its National Health Service, England has spent in the last fifteen years a third less of its resources on medical care and experiences roughly a third the expenditure

TABLE 5.2 Total Expenditures for Health Services as a Percentage of the Gross National Product, Seven Countries, Selected Periods, 1961-1973

	WHO Estimates[a]		*SSA Estimates*[b]		*McKinsey Estimates*[c]	
Country	*Year*	*Percentage of GNP*	*Year*	*Percentage of GNP*	*Year*	*Percentage of GNP*
Canada	1961	6.0	1969	7.3	1970-73	7.7
United States	1961-62	5.8	1969	6.8	1970-73	7.7
Sweden	1962	5.4	1969	6.7	1970-73	7.0
Netherlands	1963	4.8	1969	5.9	1970-73	7.3
Federal Republic of Germany	1961	4.5	1969	5.7	1970-73	6.1
France	1963	4.4	1969	5.7	1970-73	6.1
United Kingdom	1961-62	4.2	1969	4.8	1970-73	5.8

Sources: a. Brian Abel-Smith, *An International Study of Health Expenditure,* Public Paper No. 32 (Geneva: World Health Organization, 1967).
b. Joseph G. Simanis, "Medical Care Expenditure in Seven Countries," *Social Security Bulletin,* 36, (March 1973): 39.
c. Robert Maxwell, *Health Care: The Growing Dilemma,* 2nd ed. (New York: McKinsey and Company, 1975), pp. 18,68.

increase relative to GNP of Canada, Sweden, or the United States (Table 5.2).[34] To the 16 percent of Americans who favor putting doctors on salary in an English-style system, this will be a welcome argument.[35] But even to others, the experience of Great Britain suggests a financing concentration desirable in a future national health insurance program. Thus, the "conservative" emphasis on controlling inflation may best be accomplished by a greater degree of governmental centralization than even many "liberals" favor.

Of the leading U.S. plans, the Kennedy-Corman bill—with its concentrated[36] federal financing—affords the best theoretical prospects for curbing inflation. But to be effective, it must be fully implemented, and that is now unlikely. The Feldstein plan is directed at cost containment, placing financial responsibility on patients in order to restrain inflation. But to work, such a plan must discourage supplementary insurance—a daunting political task.[37] Hence, the most promising anti-inflation proposals are politically the most controversial.

CHIP or some other mixed plan is more likely, since it would offer more busines and further subsidies to health care insurers and providers without strict central budgetary control. Fiscally decentralized plans would be inflationary yet would still leave major gaps in coverage—the worst of both worlds. The more likely national health insurance programs in the coming years have modest prospects for controlling costs; a real market solution *or* effective budget ceilings have appeared too "radical" to emerge from the pulling and hauling of congressional deliberation.

Maldistribution

National health insurance is likely to be more successful in improving access than in containing costs. But financial barriers are only part of the problem. Equally serious is unavailability of care in major areas and specialties, the result of poor distribution of medical personnel.[38] No proposed remedy has worked well—neither educational loan forgiveness for service in underdoctored areas, nor substitution of rural or ghetto medical service for physicians' military obligations, nor subsidies for medical centers in underserved locales. Only a Draconian measure such as forced assignment to regions and specialties would work;[39] otherwise, young doctors have good professional and social reasons for continuing to prefer specialty practices in affluent suburban neighborhoods.

Even where specialists are present in abundance, as in metropolitan hospitals connected with university or research institutions, there may be problems of distribution of care. Other Western democracies have learned that poor distribution remains after the medical purchasing power of poor city neighborhoods (and remote rural areas) are improved. In the United States, differences in access to medical care related to income are exacerbated by racial factors. While such practices are difficult to document, there is some evidence that poor minority group patients are treated differently in facilities shared with middle-class whites, with abusive sterilization a case in point.[40]

Many observers have claimed that with the current supply of doctors, at least in primary care, there is chronic excess demand,[41] thus giving doctors much discretion. The usual "doctor-shortage" analysis is that doctors do not ration by price as much as by exercising wide choice in location; they increase queues in some places while reducing them in others by choosing interesting rather than routine work. More rationing by price may well be retarded by the doctor's sense of responsibility toward his or her patient. The physician's influence over the patients' "needs" means expanding physician supply may increase overall costs. There is no agreement on a correct strategy for dealing with the problem. One school notes that in order to avoid skyrocketing costs with national health insurance there will have to be increases in physician supply; the other argues that new doctors will expand their services to reach acceptable incomes. As a consequence, it is not surprising that none of the national health insurance proposals addresses the personnel question very forcefully.

The efficacy of the increased supply solution in dampening costs depends partly on the insurance scheme proposed; it is a more persuasive strategy where doctors and patients are both concerned about costs. It thus appears most plausible under a scheme like Feldstein's and least promising under a plan like the AMA's. HMOs also appear to offer hope that increased supplies of personnel would put downward pressure on prices (and would produce other improvements as well), but it is difficult to forecast with certainty how HMOs will fare under the various plans that encourage their formation.

Quality of Care

National health insurance, whether fiscally centralized or decentralized, is unlikely to transform the quality of medical care. It may provide incentives for preventive care,[42] but it cannot check malpractice or doubtful practice much better than present institutions do. Moreover, the enforcement of minimum "quality" standards may actually stimulate the demand for costly and inefficent procedures. The quality of medical care depends much more on professional self-regulation and consumer awareness than on any conceivable health insurance plan's regulations.

This skepticism about national health insurance's capacity to reform American medical care need not justify public policy inaction. The major aim of insurance is to avert financial disaster; other issues are peripheral to that concern. The argument that more traditional medical care will not markedly improve our health is beside the point when one asks whether the current burden of medical care expenses is sensibly distributed. Some have argued that national health insurance without incentives for prevention and improvement of health is not worth having. But would anyone seriously argue that automobile insurance, for example, is not worth having if it does not prevent accidents and improve the quality of our automobiles?

Recognizing the conflicting objectives in NHI proposals is the prerequisite for a rational debate over them. The choices include whether the United States should spend a larger share of its resources on medical care services, through the federal government or otherwise. Should efforts be made to make care more accessible (and perhaps less fancy) and of substantially higher quality (and, therefore, more expensive), and should the use of medical care be independent of ability to pay (and, therefore, likely to be more costly in the aggregate)?

The NHI debate will be a particularly obscure and frustrating one for Americans who are interested in health insurance mainly as consumers and taxpayers. First, the political rhetoric concentrates on the symbols rather than on the substance of the alternative proposals. This is nowhere more evident than in the Ford Administration's strong opposition to the Kennedy-Mills proposal, when its own plan was very similar, except that the Democratic proposal would run the necessary funds through the federal budget while the other called for the purchase of private insurance. Further, a close look at the proposals reveals important differences of values and assessments of the health care industry. If only values were at issue, one could take sides with confidence. Assessing the impact of proposed plans is more difficult, and the most diligent observers may remain confused. Finally, important problem areas in health care will not be affected by NHI.

VI. Changing Legislative Politics and the Prospects for National Health Insurance

National health insurance, though much discussed in the last half decade, has rarely proceeded to the stage of serious consideration in the U.S. legislative process. The debate, discussion, and analysis generally have expressed the exceptation that the enactment of NHI would soon follow. In practice, its function has largely been to relieve intermittently the pressure that interests groups have exerted on candidates, legislators, and presidents to take a stand on national health insurance. Since 1970 a number of different NHI bills have been regularly introduced at the beginning of each new Congress, and House and Senate sponsors have been actively recruited by supporting groups. Congress has held extensive hearings and the volume of NHI studies has sharply increased. These are important "predecisional" activities in the national policy process; issues and ideas are diffused and refined, information is generated, and supporters and opponents are mobilized. They set the substantive and political boundaries for legislative consideration when NHI becomes a legislative priority for the President and congressional leaders, and there consequently are serious attempts to move a bill through the congressional labyrinth. These activities also reveal the barriers to enactment of NHI, and a review of them prepares us to make predictions about the likely outcome of future efforts.

Throughout the late 1960s and early 1970s, the Administration and Congress dealt only sporadically with NHI. In 1974, however, it momentarily appeared that national leaders had focused their attention on the issue and that legislative action might emerge. In February, President Nixon revealed the Administration's CHIP proposal and urged congressional approval. Introduction on April 2 of a new compromise proposal by Senator Edward Kennedy and House Ways and Means Committee Chairman Wilbur Mills intensified debate over the specific features of an acceptable bill and increased the prospects for legislative action. For three months, beginning April 24, the Ways and Means Committee held extensive hearings on the major proposals. The sequence of struggles in 1974 reflects the peculiar politics of NHI amidst partisan conflict between the Congress and the Executive.

On August 5, 1974, Ways and Means began "markup" sessions on NHI legislation. After several days of staff briefings and general discussion, the committee members were presented with a "compromise" proposal drafted on Mill's instructions by the staff of the committee and HEW. It combined features of many of the major NHI bills advocated by different members of the committee during the hearings. On financing, the Kennedy-Mills bill joined the Long-Ribicoff federally financed catastrophic health program to the mandated private insurance coverage of the Nixon CHIP bill. The result was a federally financed and administered "Catastrophic Health Insurance Plan" that would be paid for by a new payroll tax, and a mandated "Employer Health Insurance Plan" that would require employers to provide their workers a standard package of *private* health insurance protection cover-g basic or noncatastrophic health expenses.

As would be expected from our analysis, the major interest groups intensely lobbied against the proposed compromise. Labor unions objected to a mandated expansion of private insurance, which would limit public financing to catastrophic coverage. Many medical groups objected to compulsory enrollment and financial regulations in both the employer and the catastrophic plans.

The Ways and Means Committee reached tentative agreement on some issues, such as the scope of insured services. On the critical issue of financing, however, the members divided along conservative/liberal lines, reflecting the ideological polarization of the interest groups. By a twelve to twelve vote the committee rejected a motion to substitute the AMA's voluntary, tax-credit approach as the compromise financing mechanism. On this vote, the five conservative southern

Democrats on the committee voted with the seven Republicans in support of the tax-credit plan. Later, the financing provisions in the mandated private insurance part of the compromise proposal were approved by a one-vote margin (twelve to eleven) on a show-of-hands vote.

On August 21, after an hour of heated discussion, Mills interrupted the debate and told the committee he had "never worked harder to reach a consensus than . . . on national health insurance. I introduced the Nixon Administration bill with Mr. Schneebeli and the compromise bill with Senator Kennedy. I think the members of the committee will agree we have done everything we can to bring about a consensus. We don't have that consensus, and I will not go to the House floor with a committee bill approved by a thirteen to twelve vote." Unable to assemble a moderate coalition from intensely committed opponents, he terminated the committee deliberations on national health insurance.

Another attempt in Congress to approve health insurance legislation occurred early in the next year. With unemployment at the highest level since 1941, there was interest in legislation providing health insurance protection for jobless workers who lost their employment-connected private health insurance.[43] Initially, the AFL-CIO, American Hospital Association, AMA, Group Health Association of America, Health Insurance Association of America, and the UAW united in support of a bill introduced by Senators Kennedy, Williams, Javits, and Schweiker. The bill would have used federal general revenues to continue the premium payments for private health insurance coverage held by unemployed workers. It would have maintained the same coverage individuals had while working for as long as they remained eligible for unemployment compensation benefits. According to a *National Journal* report, this unlikely coalition of labor unions, insurance companies, and hospitals united in support of the Kennedy bill because "it offered federal subsidies to health careproviders, new business to the insurance companies and a method for unions to protect their unemployed members."[44]

It was a short-lived coalition, however. The collapse occurred when the lobbies for the insurance industry shifted their support, preferring an alternative developed by representative Rostenkowski, chairman of the Health Subcommittee of Ways and Means. The Rostenkowski bill proposed a two-part program of temporary measures and permanent changes. The temporary provisions would continue the health insurance benefits of a newly unemployed individual. This would be financed by a temporary tax paid by insurance companies on the basis of the group health insurance premiums they collected. The permanent part of the proposal would require employers to revise their private group health insurance plans within fourteen months of enactment so that workers who lose their jobs would continue to have health insurance coverage for as long as they were eligible for unemployment compensation.

This ingenious option appeared easy to administer and it responded to the Administration's objections to any bill significantly increasing the federal budget. The permanent part of the proposal raised long-standing ideological conflicts. It mandated an expansion of the private health insurance conceptually consistent with the NHI proposals sponsored by the insurance and hospital industries, and other conservative groups. As such, the bill roused the familiar opposition of the labor unions and their NHI allies. Despite Rostenkowski's insistence that his bill was "an interim solution" that did not "commit us to any particular approach to national health insurance," many participants regarded it as a step toward national health insurance along the lines of plans supported by the insurance industry and health providers. As a result, it interjected the concerns and polarization of traditional NHI politics. The reasons given by the insurance companies for shifting their support to the Rostenkowski bill revealed the old split over government versus private financing of medical care. For example, Lawrence Cathles, Jr., a senior vice-president of Aetna Life and Casualty, stated:

> Personally, I think it [the Rostenkowski bill] is by far the best thing that has come down the pike. . . . The thing I worried

> about under the Kennedy bill was the use of government financing. . . . It would bring in another sizeable bloc of the population whose health insurance needs are paid for by the government. True, he [Kennedy] uses private insurers to administer the program, but this is not inconsistent with the position he took under the Mills-Kennedy health insurance bill. That is, a plan that places private carriers in the role of fiscal intermediaries, but it is *financed and thus controlled* entirely by the government. But the Rostenkowski approach gets away from all of that [emphasis added].[45]

Opposed to the expansion of private insurance coverage under the permanent provisions, the labor unions persuaded House Speaker Carl Albert to refer the Rostenkowski bill to the House Interstate and Foreign Commerce Committee, which had jurisdiction over the Kennedy bill. Several weeks later the Rogers subcommittee reported out a bill that retained the temporary part of the Rostenkowski bill, dropped the permanent provisions entirely, and added Medicaid coverage for jobless workers on unemployment compensation who had no health insurance while working.

At this point, the movement to enact an emergency health insurance bill for the unemployed dissipated, not because unemployment was decreasing or because any of the problems at which the bill was aimed had disappeared. It died partly because the Administration was opposed to any bill and partly because it became entangled in a jurisdictional dispute between two House committees. But primarily the bill died because the issue had shifted to the financing of NHI, and the major advocates of emergency action split over the ideological and economic concerns that have consistently polarized them.

These two attempts demonstrate that, despite some optimistic predictions, the enactment of NHI legislation in the near future is not inevitable. Because of NHI's divisiveness and cost, it will be enacted only under a special combination of economic and political circumstances. At the least, enactment will require the strong commitment and efforts of White House and congressional leaders. The likelihood of enactment, and the final form and features of a NHI bill that does make its way through the legislative process, thus depend largely upon the ideological orientation of the White House and Congress.

A mixed public/private approach, like the compromise proposal developed by the Ways and Means Committee staff in August 1974, or the Kennedy-Mills bill, would be most likely to emerge if enactment came during a period when different parties controlled the White House and Congress, or when liberals dominated one branch and conservatives the other (for example, if there were a liberal Democratic president and if the "conservative coalition" of conservative Democrats and Republicans outnumbered liberal Democrats in the Congress).[46] Under these circumstances, however, it is unlikely that agreement could be reached in Congress or between Congress and the Administration on a NHI bill, as demonstrated by the two unsuccessful attempts in the House in 1974 and 1975 to pass health insurance legislation.

Because of the strong opposition of the labor unions, enactment of something along the lines of the Nixon and Ford Administrations' CHIP proposal or the AMA Medicredit plan, which would require or encourage an expansion of private health insurance coverage, is unlikely as long as the Democrats control either the White House or Congress. A Republican president enjoyed a Republican majority in both the House and Senate during only two of the past forty-four years (1952-1953), and this is an unlikely event in the near future. Even if this were to occur, NHI probably would not be a high-priority issue. Republican political leaders in the past have supported the health industry on NHU. The AMA, health insurance companies, and hospitals have developed their NHI plans in reaction or as counterproposals to the plans supported by the unions, not with the objective of initiating legislative action.

In other words, legislative initiatives on NHI are not likely during a period of Republican control or when there is division between the White House and Congress along party or ideological lines. Serious attention to NHI and its final enactment are most likely to occur under political conditions that favor the type of government-financed NHI program supported by the unions and formalized in the Kennedy-Corman Health Security Act—that is, when there is (1) a Democratic president committed to the passage of health insurance legislation and a Democratic majority of about 295 members in the House and approximately 65 in the Senate, or (2) a sufficient Democratic majority in Congress for Democratic liberals to outnumber the coalition of conservative Democrats and Republicans. This was the political situation in 1965 when the Medicare and Medicaid programs were enacted. Marmor describes the political developments that made federal health insurance for the aged a "legislative certainty" as follows:

> The electoral outcome of 1964 guaranteed the passage of legislation on medical care for the aged. Not one of the obstacles to Medicare was left standing. In the House, the Democrats gained thirty-two new seats, giving them a more than two-to-one ratio for the first time since the heyday of the New Deal. In addition, President Johnson's dramatic victory over Goldwater could be read as a popular mandate for Medicare. The President had campaigned on the promise of social reforms—most prominently Medicare and federal aid to education—and the public seemed to have rejected decisively Goldwater's alternatives of state, local, and private initiative.
>
> Within the Congress, immediate action was taken to prevent the use of delaying tactics previously employed against both federal aid to education and medical care bills. Liberal Democratic members changed the House rules so as to reduce the power of Republican-Southern Democratic coalitions on committees to delay legislative proposals. The twenty-one-day rule was reinstated, making it possible to dislodge bills from the House Rules Committee after a maximum delay of three weeks.
>
> At the same time changes affecting the Ways and Means Committee were made which reduced the likelihood of further efforts to delay Medicare legislation. The traditional ratio of three members of the majority party to two of the minority party was abandoned for a ratio reflecting the strength of the parties in the House as a whole (two-to-one). In 1965, that meant the composition of Ways and Means shifted from fifteen Democrats and ten Republicans to seventeen Democrats and eight Repub-

> licans, insuring a pro-Medicare majority. A legislative possibility. until the election of 1964, the King-Anderson program had become a statutory certainty. The only question remaining was the precise form the health insurance legislation would take.[47]

Recent political developments are similar to those that preceded and made possible the enactment of Medicare and Medicaid. The 1974 congressional elections increased the Democratic membership in the House of Representatives from 248 to 290, reducing the strength of the "conservative coalition" (Republicans plus conservative Southern Democrats) from approximately 260 to 215. Fifty-six of the legislators who had sponsored the AMA's national health insurance proposal in the previous Congress retired or were defeated in 1974. Many of them were replaced by legislators with closer ties to labor and other liberal health groups and less inclined to embrace the AMA's or other conservative organizations' positions on NHI. In the 1976 elections, the Democrats increased their majority in the House to 292 and maintained their 1974 majority of 62 Senate seats. As shown in Table 5.3, in the 95th Congress the Democratic majority in the House of Representatives was predicted to be larger than in any previous Congress since the 1964 Congress that enacted Medicare and Medicaid.

Following the 1974 congressional elections, a number of organizational reforms were instituted in the House of Representatives with implications for NHI legislation. Junior liberal Democrats, working through the rejuvenated Democratic Caucus, deposed three committee chairmen, shifted the committee assignment authority from Ways and Means to the Steering Committee on the Caucus, required all legislative committees to have a two-to-one plus one Democratic majority, and established procedures aimed at opening committee meetings to the public and assuring freshmen better subcommittee assignments.

The Ways and Means Committee, which prior to the 94th Congress had complete jurisdiction over Medicare, Medicaid,

TABLE 5.3 Party Composition of the House and Senate: 72nd to 95th Congress

		House		Senate	
Congress	*Election Year*	*Dems.*	*Reps.*	*Dems.*	*Reps.*
72nd	1930	216	218	47	48
73rd	1932	313	117	59	36
74th	1934	322	103	69	25
75th	1936	333	89	75	17
76th	1938	262	169	69	23
77th	1940	267	162	66	28
78th	1942	222	209	57	38
79th	1944	243	190	57	38
80th	1946	188	246	45	51
81st	1948	263	171	54	42
82nd	1950	234	199	48	47
83rd	1952	213	221	47	48
84th	1954	232	203	48	47
85th	1956	234	201	49	47
86th	1958	283	154	66	34
87th	1960	263	174	64	36
88th	1962	259	176	68	32
89th	1964	295	140	67	33
90th	1966	248	187	64	36
91st	1968	243	192	58	42
92nd	1970	255	180	55	45
93rd	1972	243	192	57	43
94th	1974	290	145	62	39
95th	1976	292	143	62	39

Source: Congressional Research Service, Library of Congress.

and NHI, was changed almost beyond recognition.[48] In 1975 the size of the committee was increased from twenty-five to thirty-seven members, the Democratic majority was increased from fifteen to ten to twenty-five to twelve, and over half (nineteen) of the members in the 94th Congress were new to the committee (including four freshmen). Wilbur Mills, who had been chairman of Ways and Means since 1958, was replaced by Al Ullman (D-Oregon). Mills played a major role in the enactment of Medicare and Medicaid in 1965 and was expected to exercise major influence in the design and enactment of national health insurance legislation.

Ullman does not dominate the agenda-setting and decision-making activities of Ways and Means as did Mills. Ways and Means is not as influential in the House, or as responsive to Administration positions and proposals, as it was in the past. These chnges are due partly to the differences in personality and style of Ullman and Mills, but they are mainly due to the influx of new members in the House and the Ways and Means Committee (who do not share the chairman-dominated, consensus-oriented decision-making style under Mills), the increased Democratic majority on the committee and in the House, and the dispersion of power within Ways and Means among senior Democrats who became chairman of the newly established subcommittees.

Another important change in the House was the shift in jurisdiction over non-payroll-financed health programs and legislation from the Ways and Means Committee to the Interstate and Foreign Commerce Committee. In 1975 Ways and Means relinquished control over the Medicaid and Maternal and Child Health programs. The debate over health insurance for the unemployed raised the issue of which committee had jurisdiction over NHI but did not resolve it. National health insurance bills are being jointly referred to both committees, and the health subcommittees of both have held extensive hearings on this issue. The jurisdictional dispute provided an incentive for congressional activity on NHI during the 94th Congress, with both subcommittees eager to demonstrate their jurisdictional claims. If not resolved, the jurisdictional conflict could pose a major stumbling block to future House actions on NHI.

Congress is going to play a major role in the design of future health insurance legislation. And the size of the Democratic majority in the 95th Congress has enhanced the possibility of Congress approving a bill that expands the federal government's role in the financing of personal health care. Even with the large Democratic majority in Congress, though, the intense ideological disagreements, the economic concerns, and the polarization of the major interest groups make House and Senate approval of a NHI bill likely only if it is a high-priority item on the President's legislative agenda and if the White House provides sustained, energetic leadership in any attempt to legislate in this area.[49]

If NHI becomes a legislative priority of the President and Congress during the 95th Congress, the unions and NHI reformers will face the difficult dilemma—over which they are already divided—of whether to hold out for a complete Kennedy-Corman type of program or to support a more limited or phased-in federal program. The dilemma is that the budgetary controls and cost regulations they advocate require virtually all health expenditures to be paid by the federal government, as proposed in the Kennedy-Corman NHI bill. Because of the substantial increases in taxes and federal expenditures involved, however, it appears politically impossible to shift all privately financed health costs to the federal government at once. This has persuaded some NHI reformers to support more limited proposals like the Kennedy-Mills bill, or to support phasing in the Kennedy-Corman program by population groups or scope of benefits over a period of a year.[50] Because a mixture of private and public financing arrangements would be maintained, a reduced or staged-in federal program might severely limit the effectiveness of the cost-control mechanisms envisioned in the Kennedy-Corman proposal. In fact, steps toward a universal and comprehensive program might contribute substantially to inflation in health costs. So, while the growing concern over rising health costs has intensified support for an immediate and complete federalization of health expenditures, the budgetary impact and perceived political infeasibility of such a move has caused some to advocate a phased-in or reduced Kennedy-Corman type of federal health insurance program.

VII. Conclusion

National health insurance is again prominent on the governmental agenda. Heightened public concerns about the medical care system, in combination with Democratic domination of both the White House and Congress, make the enactment of some NHI plan likely. Yet the entrenched coalitions and ideological commitments that have historically shaped social welfare policy will continue to influence the NHI debate. The old questions—whether more federal intervention is desirable, and whether it constrains or broadens individual choice—will again be raised.

In this round of debate, as in the others, the suggestions of policy analysis and the predictions of political analysis diverge. Nowhere is this more evident than in the attempt to control medical inflation. Ironically, the "liberal" government intervention required to control costs will be opposed most vigorously by conservatives for whom cost is a central concern. For most instances of policy choice in this debate, the intervention of values and political convictions will be more subtle but equally perplexing.

Conventional political analysis suggests that middle-ground solutions are most likely to emerge. Pressures on the federal budget probably preclude immediate comprehensive federal financing of health insurance envisioned by bills like Kennedy-Corman. As a consequence, there is greater political interest in plans with high deductibles and/or compulsory employer financing of plans, which spread the costs of health insurance among several parties. Only in the event of strong and coordinated Democratic leadership zealously committed to a plan of the Kennedy-Corman type will this political prediction prove wrong.

NOTES

1. *Washington Post,* 3 April 1976, p. A3.

2. Residtributive politics are not the only type found in the health sector, Following Theodore Lowi ("American Business, Public Policy, Case

Studies, and Political Theory," *World Politics* 16 [1964]: 677-715), one can separate conflicts associated with redistributive, regultory, and distributive issues. Regulatory conflicts are about burdens and benefits affecting an industry or organized set of producers or consumers; the struggle over PSROs—professional standards review organizations—is a medical care example. Distributive questions are those we associate with "pork barrel" activities, the log-rolling and support-building that is associated with discrete allocation decisions, as, for example, in applications for Hill-Burton funds. There is clearly "politics in health" rather than a uniform "politics of health." (See Andrew B. Dunham and Theodore R. Marmor, "Political Science and Health Services Administration," paper prepared for the Association of University Programs in Health Administration, Washington, DC, September 1, 1976.) Characterizing national health insurance in redistributive terms highlights the ideological, class-struggle aspects of its politics; it does not mean that other types of political conflict are absent.

2. Edward M. Kennedy, *In Critical Condition: The Crisis in America's Health Care* (New York: Simon & Schuster, 1972).

3. "The Social Security Revolution," *Congressional Quarterly: Congress and the Nation,* Vol. 1 (Washington, DC: Congressional Quarterly Service, 1965), p. 1225.

4. This group includes Wilbur Cohen (Secretary of Health, Education, and Welfare, 1968-1969); I. S. Falk (Social Security Administration; 1936-1954); Robert Ball (Commissioner of the Social Security Administration, 1962-1973); and Nelson Cruikshank (Advisory Council Social Security Financing, 1957-1958/Health Insurance Benefits Advisory Council, 1965-1972).

5. T. R. Marmor, *The Politics of Medicare* (Chicago: Aldine, 1973), p. 111.

6. Murray Edelman, *The Symbolic Uses of Politics* (Chicago: University of Illinois Press, 1964), pp. 29, 125, 134-138, 160-161.

7. Richard Nixon, "The Nation's Health Care System," *Weekly Compilation of Presidential Documents,* vol. 5, no. 28, July 10, 1969, p. 963.

8. Kennedy, *In Critical Condition.*

9. "Our Ailing Medical System," *Fortune,* January 1970.

10. George Meany, statement of the AFL-CIO, *Hearings on National Health Insurance,* Committee on Ways and Means, 11 vols., October-November 1971, p. 239.

11. Ronald Andersen et al., "The Public's View of the Crisis in Medical Care: An Impetus for Changing Delivery Systems?" *Economic and Business Bulletin* 24 (Fall, 1971): 44-52. See also Aaron Wildavsky, "Doing Better and Feeling Worse," Working Paper No. 19, Graduate School of Public Policy, University of California, Berkeley, March 1975, p. 2. The salience of the health care issue is increasing. Between 1972 and 1975 the proportion of those who regarded health care as a critical problem increased from 42 to 55 percent. Fifty-five percent of the respondents ranked health care as a "very, very important" issue (5 on a 5-point scale) compared to 42 percent three years ago. See remarks by Dorothy Lynch in

National Health Council, *A Declaration of Interdependence: Developing America's Health Policy,* Proceedings of the Twenty-Fourth Annual National Health Forum, March 16-17, 1976, Philadelphia, Pennsylvania, p. 36.

12. Stephen P. Strickland, *U.S. Health Care: What's Right and What's Wrong,* (New York: Universe Books, 1972), pp. 43, 102.

13. Council on Wage and Price Stability, *The Problem of Rising Health Care Costs,* no. 81 (Washington, DC, The Bureau of National Affairs, Inc., April 26, 1976), pp. x-4.

14. Michael Meyer, *Catastrophic Illnesses and Catastrophic Health Insurance* (Washington, DC: The Heritage Foundation, Inc., 1974), p. 4. Fewer than 1 percent spend more than $5000 a year on medical care.

15. U.S. Executive Office of the President, *Budget of the United States Government 1976: Special Analysis* (Washington, DC: Government Printing Office, 1975), p. 170; U.S. Congress, House of Representatives, Committee on Ways and Means, *Basic Charts on Health Care* (Washington, DC: Government Printing Office, July 8, 1975), pp. 44-45.

16. L. B. Russell et al., *Federal Health Spending: 1969-74* (Washington, DC: National Planning Association, 1974), pp. 62, 64.

17. Only some 70,000 of the 295,000 practicing in the country are pediatricians or general practitioners, *Profiles of Medical Practice, 1974,* reference edition (Chicago: American Medical Practice, 1974), pp. 95, 100.

18. *Medical World News,* February 23, 1976, p. 25.

19. See, for example, Brian Abel-Smith, "Value for Money in Health," *Social Security Bulletin* 37 (July 1974): 18.

20. See, for example, Barbara Ehrenrich and John Ehrenrich, *The American Health Empire: Power, Profit and Politics* (New York: Random House, 1970); and Rick Carlson, *The End of Medicine* (New York: John Wiley, 1975).

21. Ronald Wilson and Elijah White, "Changes in Morbidity, Disability, and Utilization Differentials Between the Poor and the Nonpoor, Data from the Health Interview Survey: 1964 and 1973." Paper presented at the 102nd Annual Meeting of the American Public Health Association, October 21, 1974, cited in Dorothy Rice and Douglas Wilson, "The American Medical Economy: Problems and Perspectives," *Journal of Health Politics, Policy and Law* 1 (Summer 1976): 160.

22. See Michael Meyer, "Catastrophic Illnesses."

23. Martin Feldstein, "A New Approach to National Health Insurance," *The Public Interest* 23 (Spring 1971). This is only one version of Feldstein's MRI. See the discussion later in this chapter.

24. See note to Figure 5.1.

25. Waldman, *National Health Insurance,* pp. 16, 161; John Holahan, *Financing Health Care for the Poor,* pp. 86-90.

26. AMA Statement on National Health Insurance (by Dr. Max Parrot), *Hearings on National Health Insurance,* Ways and Means Committee, October-November, 1971, p. 1951.

27. Ibid.

28. Feldstein, "A New Approach."

29. In addition to medical inflation (point 4), Feldstein is concerned about the impact of increased taxes, fearing that national income may be lowered. Consumer's Union (CU) warns that "most cost estimates are unreliably partisan" and implies that the only important issue is "new spending for medical care." In doing this, CU is technically in error and could be accused of misleading its readers—additional costs to result from giving things away "free" and paying for them with tax revenue. Just as a tax on cigarettes changes their price relative to other things and presumably how many of them are purchased. So too does an increase in the tax upon work—either a payroll or an income tax—change the terms upon which work is traded for leisure. Nevertheless, the distortion of the supply of work effort engendered by the taxes necessary to finance the very substantial difference in federal expense between Feldstein's proposed major risk insurance, perhaps $10 billion, and the much higher federal price tag of a scheme like Kennedy-Griffiths or Kennedy-Mills is not known. CU, and the public, might thus be forgiven for being more concerned about other issues (concerning power and choice mechanisms) connected with running health insurance monies through the federal budget, than with its distortion of work-leisure choices.

30. The term, of course, is that of John Kenneth Galbraith in his *New Industrial State* (Boston: Houghton Mifflin, 1967). Few economists were persuaded of the substantial area of autonomy for most of the industrial sector which characterizes Galbraith's presentation. It appears never to have been pointed out, however, that medicine may be the one major industry in which the "revised sequence"—the virtual determination of demand by producers—is more than a myth.

31. Douglas Conrad and Theodore Marmor, "Private Health Insurance Supplementation Under NHI," unpublished manuscript, February 1977.

32. Rashi Fein, *The Doctor Shortage* (Washington, DC: Brookings, Ch. 1. 1967).

33. See Odin Anderson, *Health Care: Can There Be Equity?* (New York: John Wiley, 1973) for evidence on postwar price and expenditure trends in England, Sweden, and the United States. A recently published work, *National Health Insurance: Can We Learn From Canada?* ed. Spyros Andreopoulos (New York: John Wiley, 1975) documents the financing role of public authorities in Canada and their frustration over the past decade in curbing expenditure and price increases to anything below that of the United States. See particularly Chapter 3 by R. G. Evans. See also T. R. Marmor, C. A. Wittman, and T. C. Heagy, "Politics, Public Policy, and Inflation," in *Health: A Victim or Cause of Inflation,* ed. M. Zubkoff (New York: Milbank Memorial Fund, 1975). Gordon R. Trapnell Associates, "A Comparison of the Costs of the Major National Health Insurance Proposals" (DHEW, October 1976, mineo) is a careful prediction of both social and governmental costs under proposed plans. Costs will go up even without an NHI program; public sector expenditures would be decreased by the AMA proposal; any of the others would increase them. For example, with no NHI program, government expenditures will be $84.5 billion by 1980; under Long-Ribicoff the projection is $97.7; under Health

Security, $200.9. Differences in total cost are less striking: $233.5 billion with no plan, $248.5 billion under the AHA (most expensive) plan. Costs to individuals are smallest under HSA ($38.2 billion); greatest if no NHI is enacted ($70.1 billion).

34. See T. Marmor, T. Heagy, and N. Hoffman, "National Health Insurance: Some Lessons from the Canadian Experience," *Policy Sciences* (special issue on comparative policy research) 6 (December 1975): 447-466. More specifically on inflation controls, see Marmor, Wittman, and Heagy, "Politics, Public Policy, and Medical Inflation."

35. D. Lynch, National Health Council, *Declaration of Independence,* p. 35.

36. By "concentration" we mean a single unit of government paying the bill—the Health Security Board in the case of Kennedy-Corman. By contrast, our present medical financing is dispersed among patients, numerous insurance carriers, and federal, state, and local government agencies.

37. Interviews with HEW officials suggest that any effort to *change* the current tax advantages of health insurance meet with fierce resistance. This resistance led Stuart Altman, Deputy Assistant Secretary for Health, Office of Planning and Evaluation, HEW, to conclude that more drastic constraints on insurance would have a near-zero probability of enactment.

38. See, among others, the comments by Michael Zubkoff in The National Health Council, *Declaration of Independence,* p. 62.

39. No absolute minimum ratio of doctors to patients has ever been agreed upon, and the notion of geographic equality—at whatever the national average—is not sensible because there will always be heavy concentrations of personnel at regional medical centers.

40. See U.S. Congress, House Committee on Ways and Means, *National Health Insurance, Panel Discussion,* before the subcommittee on health, July 10, 11, 17, 24 and September 12, 1975, 94th Congress, 1st Session (Washington, DC: Government Printing Office, 1975). For intraurban differences, see David Kotelchuck, ed., *Prognosis Negative: Crisis in the Health Care System* (New York: Vintage Books, 1976), Chapters 1, 2.

41. Rashi Fein, *The Doctor Shortage;* Martin Feldstein, "The Rising Price of Physicians' Services," *Review of Economics and Statistics* 52 (May 1970).

42. It should be noted that there is little evidence to support the general enthusiasm for preventive care. There are indications that primary prevention—for example, prenatal care—effectively prevents some maternal, infant, and child problems. But there is evidence that mass screening programs and even the annual physical checkups are economically wasteful and only occasionally detect conditions that are aided by early treatment. Economists Burton Weisbrod and Ralph Andreano conclude that preventive care can increase costs without significantly raising the level of health. Apparent cost savings in Kaiser-Permanente (which is often cited as a model of the medical and financial efficacy of prevention) they attribute to "various factors, many of which are unrelated to preventive care." See Ralph Andreano and Burton Weisbrod, *American Health Policy & Perspective and Choices* (Chicago: Rand McNally, 1974), p. 35.

43. See John K. Iglehart, "Health Report/Jobless Medical Aid Debate Focuses on Financing Method," *National Journal Reports,* March 29, 1975, pp. 457-463; Iglehart. "Health Report/Feuding, Ford Opposition Peril Jobless Health Insurance," *National Journal Reports,* April 19, 1975, pp. 592-594; Iglehart, "Health Report/Speaker Supports Rogers in Dispute with Ways and Means," *National Journal Report,* May 24, 1975, p. 773; *Congressional Quarterly Weekly Report* (Washington, DC: Congressional Quarterly Service, 1975), pp. 537-540, 608-609, 769-770, 809-810, 879-880, 927-928, 1034, 1091-1095.

44. Iglehart, "Jobless Medical Aid Debate Focuses on Financing Method," p. 458.

45. Ibid., pp. 462-463.

46. John F. Manley, *The Politics of Finance: The House Committee on Ways and Means,* (Boston: Little, Brown, 1973), especially pp. 16-22.

47. Marmor, *The Politics of Medicare,* pp. 59-60.

48. See Manley, *The Politics of Finance;* Richard F. Fenno, Jr., *Congressmen in Committees* (Boston: Little, Brown, 1973); M. Kenneth Bowler, "The New Committee on Ways and Means: Policy Implications of Recent Changes in the House Committee," paper prepared for delivery at the 1976 Annual Meeting of the American Political Science Association, Chicago, September 2-5, 1976.

49. See Marmor, *The Politics of Medicare;* James L. Sundquist, *Politics and Policy* (Washington, DC: Brookings, 1968); and M. Kenneth Bowler, *The Nixon Guaranteed Income Proposal* (Cambridge: Ballinger, 1974), pp. 123-173.

50. This direction in national policy had not gained significant political support as of this writing; thus, it is not considered in the text. See the discussion of the Scheur (Child Health Care) bill by Theodore Marmor and Wilbur Cohen before the Health Subcommittee of the House Committee on Interstate and Foreign Commerce, Washington, DC, June 16, 1976.

Chapter 6

Reducing Hospital Capacity
Public Sector Options

> Consistently where social problems arise because of distorted private incentives, we try to impose a solution without remedying the incentive structure. And, equally consistently, the power of the incentive structure defeats us.[8]

The reduction of hospital capacity in the United States has become a major health policy goal because excess hospital capacity is widely believed to contribute to excessive increases in hospital costs. The National Health Policy Planning Guidelines (DHEW, 1975) contain a planning standard of 4.0 hospital beds per 1000 persons as a maximum, accompanied by an 80 percent occupancy rate for short-term community hospitals. When the guidelines were adopted the United States was experiencing 4.5 hospital beds per 1000, with a 75 percent occupany rate. Therefore, these guidelines imply that a substantial reduction in existing hospital capacity is desirable.

In this chapter, we evaluate the most widely discussed public sector options for reducing hospital capacity. We conclude that the case for closing hospitals through direct public sector action is weak. Instead, we favor public sector actions

Authors' Note: *From Jon B. Christianson and Walter McClure, "On Public Sector Options for Reducing Hospital Capacity,"* Journal of Health and Human Resources Administraton, *Vol. 4, No. 1 (Summer 1981), pp. 73-91. Reprinted by permission. The research upon which this chapter is based was funded by a grant from the McNight Foundation, St. Paul, Minnesota.*

aimed at changing the incentives of decision makers so that they incur financial penalties for supporting excess capacity. Since this incentive-based approach could prove relatively unattractive politically, it requires a carefully staged implementation to be successful. In the concluding section of the chapter we propose a sequence of public sector actions that we believe could reduce hospital capacity primarily by changing private incentives.

Nature of the Problem

Throughout this chapter we will use the term "hospital capacity" in reference not only to numbers of hospital beds, but also to the variable inputs, such as labor and equipment, associated with these beds. Therefore we define "excess hospital capacity" as hospital beds, equipment, and labor unnecessary for the effective provision of medical care to a given population. Our definition includes both underutilized capacity and needlessly utilized capacity.

The present concern about excess hospital capacity derives from a concern about hospital costs. Of the 400 percent increase in per capita hospital costs between 1960 and 1974, the proportion attributable to excess hospital capacity is a matter of debate.[2] Some estimates place the cost of an unused hospital bed at 50 percent of the cost of an occupied bed, while other estimates are in the range of 8-10 percent.[3] The difference in estimates reflects different assumptions about the relationship between staffing and hospital occupancy. Estimates of the cost of excess capacity are complicated by a second consideration. Hospital use often seems to be related more to the availability of hospital capacity than to objective measures of the health status of the patient population. Therefore it has been argued that reducing hospital capacity can lower hospitalization expenditures by reducing unnecessary hospitalization of patients.

Taking these two factors into account, McClure has estimated that roughly 20 percent of the nation's hospital capacity could be retired with no threat to health but with a potential savings of over $6 billion annually.[4] Since a reduction in capacity could reduce hospital costs with no apparent adverse impact on health, the widespread existence of excess capacity deserves explanation. We believe that it can be explained quite reasonably as a result of faulty incentives facing hospital decision makers.

About 90 percent of hospital expenditures are paid for through private insurers, Medicaid, and Medicare. The capital and operating costs associated with excess capacity are included in the charges of hospitals and therefore in the determination of private insurance premiums. Employers pay for private insurance through negotiated contributions to employee health benefit plans. While excess hospital capacity directly increases the necessary employer contribution, the employer probably is able to pass a portion of this cost "forward" to the consumer in the form of higher product prices, and a portion "backward" to the employee in the form of smaller wage increases. Moreover, since the costs of excess hospital capacity are only a small part of the costs of production for any employer, their impact on unit product prices and/or the wages of a single employee is marginally small.

Hospital reimbursements made by government through the Medicaid and Medicare programs are based on reported costs, which include the costs of excess capacity. Government finances these expenditures on hospital care through tax revenues. Therefore, excess hospital capacity requires the collection of otherwise unnecessary tax monies or a diversion of funds from other areas of public expenditure. Again, the impact at the individual level of supporting excess capacity through higher taxes or lower levels of other public services is small.

Because the costs of excess hospital capacity to any single resident are likely to be inconsequential, few individuals would find it rational to devote time and effort to the reduction of the excess on the sole basis of personal economic gain. Also, the costs of excess capacity in any given community are partially funded by nonresidents of that community, through payment of federal and state taxes and through purchase of insurance premiums based on areawide, rather than local, hospital costs. On the other hand, the benefits of excess capacity remain concentrated in the community. It has been argued that hospital administrators and trustees receive job satisfaction in direct proportion to the size of their hospitals.[5] Excess hospital capacity can mean more jobs in the community and can help in attracting physician staff; it permits physicians to schedule their patients more conveniently, to hospitalize more patients, and consequently to increase incomes. Furthermore, a large, full-service hospital can be a source of civic pride and, particularly in rural areas, a symbol of the economic viability of a community even when underoccupied. In summary, the benefits of excess capacity are highly visible and tend to be concentrated locally, while the costs are relatively hidden, small to any single individual and partially borne by nonresidents of the community. This imbalance creates a strong economic incentive for the development of excess hospital capacity on a community-by-community basis.

In attempting to deal with this problem, the public sector has two broad options. The faulty and misleading incentives that now exist can be accepted as a "fact of life," and attempts can be made to eliminate excess hospital capacity as it develops. This we will call the "direct" approach to capacity reduction. It concentrates directly on altering an end product, which in this case is hospital capacity. Alternatively, actions can be taken to change the prevailing incentives of decision makers so that they are rewarded for the reduction of excess hospital capacity. This strategy, which we will call the "indirect" approach, assumes that by changing the incentives in the process that yielded excess capacity, the excess capacity itself can be eliminated. The closure of specific hospitals through regulatory authority would be a "direct" approach to capacity reduction, while a restructuring of the market for hospital services to penalize hospitals that maintain excess capacity would be an "indirect" strategy.

The Allocation of Resources to Hospital-Capacity Reduction

Given that different options are available for public sector action, but that public sector resources are limited, it becomes important to allocate these resources among different strategies so that they achieve the greatest possible impact. In making resource-allocation decisions, it is commonly agreed that additional resources should be devoted to the pursuit of a particular goal in a particular manner only as long as the benefits generated exceed the costs of the resources employed. The primary difficulty in applying this rule to the reduction of hospital capacity involves the definition and measurement of the appropriate marginal benefits and costs. However, even a general discussion of this criterion can be useful in comparing the relative potential of direct and indirect hospital-capacity reduction efforts.[6]

For convenience of discussion, assume that the gains and losses from hospital-capacity reduction can be converted to dollar amounts, at least conceptually, and that only one action to reduce capacity is available. We will call the resources devoted to that activity "units of effort." The value of devoting public sector resources to hospital-capacity reduction is uncertain, depending on both the probability that a public sector policy will succeed in reducing capacity (given the circumstances of its implementation) and the value of the capacity that would be reduced. The product of the probability that a reduction will occur and its ultimate value is defined as the expected value of a unit of effort devoted to capacity reduction. The relationship between effort expended on reducing hospital capacity and its expected value probably will be positive for most of the resources allocated to capacity reduction by the public sector. It also seems probable that continued expansion of public sector efforts to reduce capacity eventually will yield diminishing returns. That is, the total value of the reduced hospital capacity will increase, but at a decreasing rate, as additional public sector resources are devoted to this activity. This seems reasonable since efforts to reduce capacity that have the highest expected values probably will be undertaken first.

Each community, or hospital service area, will face a different productivity relationship between effort expanded and the expected dollar value of the capacity which that effort will eliminate. In areas of great excess capacity, a sensitized public, and/or relatively acquiescent hospitals, the expected dollar value of a unit of effort expended in hospital-capacity reduction may be high. The expected value of the same effort may be much lower in communities where these or similar circumstances are absent. However, in each community the expected marginal benefits from devoting incremental amounts of effort to hospital-capacity reduction will decline as total effort increases.

In determining their appropriate level of public sector effort, communities also must consider the costs of that effort. Since the time and abilities of individuals have alternate uses, as do any dollars devoted to hospital-capacity reduction, resources will have to be drawn away from increasingly higher-valued alternative public sector projects as capacity-reduction efforts are increased. Therefore, the marginal costs of reducing hospital capacity increase as total effort increases. These marginal costs also will vary by community. For instance, if the productivity of resources devoted to health promotion and education is large in a particular locale, a great deal must be given up when these resources are used in capacity-reduction activities instead. Thus, the marginal (opportunity) costs of hospital-capacity-reduction efforts are high in this community. Using the equalization of marginal costs and benefits as a decision rule, there is an optimal (different) level of effort that should be devoted to hospital-capacity reduction in every community. Effort in excess of this level may still yield positive benefits, but it is not rational public policy. The resources required to accomplish further capacity reduction at some point could be more effectively utilized in other activities.

When there are many possible approaches to capacity reduction, each with different marginal benefits and costs, the total public sector resources available for capacity reduction and other objectives should be apportioned among the various activities so that marginal benefits per dollar of marginal cost are equal for each activity. The exact nature of the optimal allocation will depend on the marginal benefits and costs for all activities and therefore will vary from community to community. It is possible that devoting effort to two activities simultaneously could maximize net benefits if the marginal benefits of one capacity-reduction activity are partially dependent on the amount of effort expended in another. Any rational overall policy should exploit such interdependencies so long as the marginal benefit-marginal cost decision rule is not violated.

In summary, the appropriate level of effort to devote to any single hospital-capacity-reduction activity depends on (1) the probability that that activity actually will result in hospital-capacity reduction; (2) the value of the hospital capacity that it would eliminate, measured primarily by operating dollars required to maintain the excess capacity prior to elimination; and (3) the value of the outcome which would result if the same effort were devoted to other capacity-reduction activities or to other public sector goals. This implies that relatively few resources should be devoted in aggregate to a hospital-capacity-reduction activity that (1) has a low probability of affecting change, or (2) will produce changes of little value, or (3) has a high opportunity cost in terms of promising alternative activities foregone.

The Direct Capacity-Reduction Strategy

The three criteria developed above can be used to evaluate "direct" public sector approaches to capacity reduction. The two most commonly discussed direct approaches are certificate-of-need (CON) review and appropriateness review.[7]

Under the CON provisions of the National Health Planning and Resources Development Act, health system agencies (HSAs) can recommend approval or disapproval of any hospital action that would increase total bed capacity, alter services provided by the institution, or entail an expenditure of over $100,000 for equipment. By disapproval, a local HSA (subject to review at the state level) can "freeze" a community's hospital capacity on the presumption that population growth eventually will bring hospital usage and capacity within the desired guidelines. Using CON review, an HSA can "target" individual hospitals for closure by refusing all of their requests for equipment purchase and modernization. This can make the hospital less attractive to its physician staff, cause physicians to place patients in other hospitals, and eventually destroy the continued viability of the targeted hospital.

The appropriateness-review provisions of the act can be employed to much the same effect. HSAs are authorized periodically to review the appropriateness of individual hospitals within the context of the area's health care system. A judgment that a particular hospital is "inappropriate" would carry no direct sanctions under the present provisions of the act, but the hospital would no doubt be stigmatized by such a ruling. It would find its community support reduced and would encounter greater difficulty in recruiting physician staff. Over time this could result in a decline in patient census and closure or merger with a more viable institution.

Since both CON and appropriateness reviews depend on a gradual attrition of hospital capacity, they would not provide quick results.[8] Consequently there has been some legislative interest expressed in changing the nature of appropriateness review from a planning to a regulatory activity.[9] A negative appropriateness review in this context would be sufficient to close a hospital. In addition, as exemplified by New York State, authority to close hospitals can be acquired through legislation at the state level.

Likelihood of Success

There are two considerations that lead to a low assessment of the probability that HSAs or other public sector agencies can achieve a signficant reduction in hospital beds using the instruments described above. First, there are several groups that suffer important losses when a hospital is closed: the administrator, hospital employees, physician staff, hospital volunteer groups, trustees, and the hospital's ethnic, religious, or locational constituency, to name the more obvious. They will strongly resist public sector efforts to close their hospitals. The gainers, as discussed previously, benefit relatively little on an individual basis (even though collective savings may be substantial) and therefore have only weak incentives to support closure activities. Thus, the faulty economic incentives that contribute to excess capacity make efforts to reduce that capacity politically unattractive. By pursuing hospital-capacity reduction, HSAs risk the loss of important political constituencies, and cannot be assured that their actions will win the support of any other organized groups. Assuming that HSAs in most communities are concerned with establishing a base of community support, but are somewhat risk-averse (a quality that Enthoven[10] believes to be characteristic of public sector decision makers in general), it seems likely that they would attempt to avoid a lengthy battle for capacity reduction. In the same vein, Valdeck[11] argues that most HSA decisions will reflect the interests of providers and narrowly defined consumer groups, rather than the diffuse interests of the whole community.

A second problem that will complicate the capacity-reduction efforts of public agencies is the necessity for them to identify *individual* hospitals with "unnecessary" capacity. Approximate measures of excess hospital capacity can be constructed on a community basis, but no irrefutable criteria exist in principle to determine whether one hospital in the community has unnecessary capacity relative to another. Consequently, although the legal authority probably exists to close hospitals,[12] direct regulatory attempts to do so would likely result in "protracted and very expensive litigation . . . and the outcome will seldom be certain until the final appeals are exhausted."[13] The outcome of such litigation would depend on the ability of public agencies to refute charges of prejudicial behavior in targeting specific hospitals for closure. Lacking clearly defensible criteria for identifying unnecessary capacity on a hospital-by-hospital basis, and characterized by a degree of risk-averseness, public agencies will seek to avoid litigation and therefore will be constrained in their ability to promote capacity reduction.

Value of Capacity Reduced

Even if the public sector did succeed in reducing hospital capacity through direct action, there are several reasons to expect that the actual benefits (as measured by the dollar savings from the capacity eliminated) would be relatively small. First, it seems probable that only relatively low-cost hospitals would be affected. If HSAs or other public sector agencies moved to close hospitals, Altman[14] argues, providers would not be united in their opposition. When a particular hospital is closed or its capacity reduced, other hospitals stand to gain through increased patient loads and higher revenues. Consequently, hospitals may devote their lobbying efforts to the protection of only their individual interests. In this regard, one would expect larger hospitals to be the most successful, since they have larger, more sophisticated planning staffs and more resources to devote to influencing the judgments of regulators and planners. In the process of targeting hospitals for closure through direct public action, smaller, less affluent hospitals probably would be the losers. But only a very small portion of total hospital costs are generated in these small hospitals: Consider that 50 percent of the hospitals in the United States account for only 10 percent of total hospital expenditures, while 12 percent of the hospitals account for one-half of all expenditures. The closure of small hospitals apparently would contribute in only a minor way to a reduction of hospital costs nationwide.

The likely benefits from direct, public sector efforts at capacity reduction become more problematical if the current targets of 4.0 beds per 100 and an 80 percent occupancy rate are used to guide decisions. Part of the difficulty in using these guidelines to make and defend hospital closure decisions is found in the geographical diversity of the health care system.[15] A second potential problem is that the guidelines focus narrowly on hospital bed supply and ignore other inputs in the production of hospital services. Even if bed supply were reduced, the impact on hospital expenditures would not be substantial unless other aspects of hospital capacity (labor, materials, and the like) were reduced commensurately. (A more appropriate focus would be community per capita hospital expense, as we explain later in this chapter.) Thus, while the guidelines now appear to be deceptively simple, their effectiveness in the containment of hospital costs in practice seems questionable.

In summary, it appears doubtful that the expected benefits of direct public sector attempts to reduce hospital capacity would be great: The probability of closing larger, more costly, more politically powerful hospitals through public sector action is small. There is a higher probability that smaller, politically weaker hospitals can be closed, but the benefits from doing so are small.

Cost

As is clear from the above discussion, the public sector would have to devote considerable effort toward the elimination of hospital beds through direct methods in order to attain a reasonable chance of success. This required effort would increase rapidly as the more obvious examples of excess capacity are eliminated. Staff time and funds would be required to evaluate hospitals, mollify interest groups, hold hearings, and research legal questions. If an affected hospital were to institute a lawsuit, there would be a further drain on the resources of governmental agencies. However, as Frankenhoff[16] observes, "The actual level of federal resources available to the newly designated HSA is low, some would argue too low for effective fulfillment of its mission," and "existing health planning manpower is inadequate." This limitation on resources suggests a high opportunity cost associated with direct hospital-capacity-reduction efforts by HSAs. An extensive allocation of resources to capacity reduction would detract from the ability of HSAs to pursue other important health priorities set forth in the planning act (for example, the provision of primary care to underserved areas, development of group practices and HMOs, increasing utilization of physician assistants, disease prevention, and health promotion).

With or without a lawsuit, the closure of hospitals would generate intense political pressure for public sector compensation of the injured parties (Schultze[17] calls this characteristic of public sector action the "do no direct harm principle"). Compensatory actions might include unemployment and job relocation benefits for displaced employees, reimbursement of the equity value of the closed facility, and/or financial aid for the adaptation of the facility to an alternate use. Local and state governments would have difficulty resisting this pressure, and any calculation of the cost of capacity reduction would have to include their expenditures along with the value of HSA efforts in alternative uses.

Summary

On the basis of the considerations developed above, we do not believe that it is rational policy for the public sector to devote more than minimal effort to direct hospital-capacity-reduction activities, if this strategy is pursued in isolation. This conclusion is buttressed by the experience of other nations, where even virtually complete government authority to eliminate capacity has been successfully exercised only when government has experienced extreme financial pressure.[18]

An Incentive-Oriented Strategy

The conclusions of the previous section suggest that the public sector should explore alternatives to direct methods for reducing hospital capacity. We are aware of at least two indirect, incentive-oriented strategies with the potential to be effective: (1) the incorporation into present reimbursement systems of a "penalty" for excess capacity, and (2) the reorganization of the market for hospital services to increase the general cost-consciousness of administrators and physicians. We briefly describe these strategies below, before suggesting a course of action for the public sector, and in particular for health systems agencies.

Reimbursement Penalties

Some state-sponsored programs review hospital charges to incorporate penalties for underutilized beds and services into hospital reimbursement rates. For hospitals or hospital departments with low occupancy rates, reimbursements are set below reported costs on the premise that these costs reflect expenses incurred in maintaining excess capacity. Theoretically, hospitals are rewarded for eliminating excess capacity, since this allows them to escape the reimbursement penalty.

In practice, reimbursement penalties appear to have the greatest effect when physicians have relatively little discretion in determining the demand for hospital services.[19] However, the likelihood that reimbursement penalties can be implemented successfully on a wider scale is questionable. The use of occupancy rates as guidelines for identifying excess capacity introduces incentives for cost-increasing behavior; in areas where staff physicians have greater discretionary power, they can aid "their" hospitals in escaping rate penalties by hospitalizing more patients. Administrators can do the same by relaxing utilization-review procedures. Both actions would drive up occupancy rates and increase the hospital's reimburseable charges but also would result in higher community per capita hospital expenses. (Many of the problems associated with the use of occupancy rates to guide reimbursements could be avoided by instituting a ceiling on areawide hospital expenditures, as described in the concluding section of the chapter.)

Reorganizing the Market for Hospital Services

A second indirect approach to capacity reduction which the public sector might adopt is the stimulation of cost-conscious competition in the provision of hospital services. One mechanism for accomplishing this objective is the establishment of "health care plans."[20] A health care plan can be informally defined as any organization that (1) provides (or arranges to provide) a specified set of medical services (when medically appropriate) to a defined set of voluntarily enrolled consumers, where (2) the set of providers in the organization does not constitute more than some fixed percentage (say 50 percent) of practicing physicians in a medical service area, and where (3) the basic mode of payment for services by enrollees is a fixed periodic premium or capitation payment (with no limitations on the manner in which providers are reimbursed).[21] The health maintenance organization is one possible form of health care plan, but there are other organizations that would fit this definition as well.

In contrast to the incentives created by present insurance coverage (where consumer premiums are not related to the provider chosen), providers organized as a health care plan would be rewarded for cost-consciousness. In order to remain within its predetermined budget and to attract customers from standard insurance plan options, a health care plan would have to offer competitive premiums. Therefore it would try to avoid unnecessary use of the hospital and to choose cost-effective hospitals for placing patients. Hospitals that are not overbuilt and have not purchased excessive equipment would be attractive to cost-conscious health care plans. In areas where the development of health care plans was extensive and competition among them and between plans and traditional providers was keen, inefficient, overbuilt hospitals would be unable to attract health care plan patients. Furthermore, as insurers lost subscribers to health care plans and physicians lost patients, both would have incentives to put pressure on hospitals to reduce costs. Thus, even those hospitals without health care plan patients would have new incentives to maintain facilities of an efficient size. Hospitals unable or unwilling to respond to these pressures would find their unused capacity increasing and ultimately would face closure or merger.

The incentives competitive health care plans would create would address directly the implicit objective of hospital-capacity reduction—the control of per capita hospital expenses. Since health care plans would change physician incentives for excessive hospitalization of patients, their development theoretically could stimulate not only the elimination of existing empty beds, but also the reduction of excessive physician-induced hospital use and the capacity required for it.

The community that best demonstrates the practicality of this approach is Minneapolis-St. Paul, where there are seven competing HMOs.[22] In order to control premium increases and attract enrollees, the HMOs have reduced the utilization of hospital services by their enrollees. This has affected hospitals in the Twin Cities in two ways: It has reduced the demand for hospital beds on a systemwide basis, and it has redistributed patients away from hospitals with no HMO affiliation.

Using conservative assumptions, we estimate that the lower hospitalization of HMO enrollees has reduced the need for hospital beds in the Twin Cities by approximately 220 beds (out of a total of 10,000) in the last five years. We can also project conservatively a reduction in bed demand of 550 *additional* beds in the next four years.[23] This does not represent an *addition* to excess hospital capacity in the community, since by our definition hospital beds unnecessarily utilized were already in excess. Rather it is a translation of excess capacity into a more visible form, which is also less expensive to the community if accompanied by some cutback in hospital staff. Besides their impact on total area hospitalization, the HMOs have redistributed the demand for hospital care among hospitals. While the majority of Twin Cities hospitals have experienced lower occupancy rates because of HMO growth, a minority with HMO affiliations have benefited.

Because an HMO affiliation can increase occupancy rates, several Twin Cities hospitals have actively pursued HMO business. They have done this by offering special financial arrangements to HMOs. The two largest HMOs have negotiated discounted rates with area hospitals, while the smaller HMOs have been successful in developing different arrangements, including risk-sharing with hospitals. These contractual relationships and negotiated rates between HMOs and hospitals in the Twin Cities have had two important effects on the hospital system. First, the hospitals seeking to attract or retain HMO business have had to become increasingly cost-conscious. Partially because of hospital-rate review in Minnesota, it is difficult for hospitals to subsidize HMO discounts by increasing their rates for other patients. Therefore, in hospitals where discounts are given HMO enrollees, there are strong incentives for the development of cost-effective management techniques. Second, HMOs have tended to form their primary affiliations with relatively low-cost, "front-line" hospitals, because these facilities do not contain expensive, underutilized specialty departments and equipment that must be subsidized through general patient charges. If HMO enrollment continues to grow, it apparently will contribute to the development of a hospital system characterized by many relatively basic, front-line hospitals and only a few larger medical centers providing the full range of specialty services. In summary, although the impact of HMO membership growth on the incentives of hospital decision makers in Minneapolis-St. Paul is still in the embryonic stage, the initial developments appear promising.

The Politics of Incentive-Based Strategies

The public sector could encourage the development of health care plans and their competition with traditional providers by public endorsements, educational efforts, start-up grants and loans, legislation of market entry conditions, and legal actions. However, past experience with government promotion of incentive-based policies in general and HMO development in particular is not encouraging. The passage of the Federal HMO Act (1973) was preceded by a major public relations-educational effort. As a direct result of this effort, and prior to passage of the legislation itself, a large number of new HMOs were formed and a great deal of interest was generated in HMO development. Subsequent to passage of the act, interest in HMOs declined and so did their rate of formation. In return for developmental grants and mandated employer access, the HMO Act required "a relatively broad range of minimum services, a relatively narrow range of organizational characteristics, and an added burden of administrative expense."[24] Starr[25] concludes that "while presumably aimed at making a less costly form of health care available, it [the HMO Act[seemed to do everything possible to make that alternative more immediately expensive to the consumer." The provisions of the HMO Act reflect a general characteristic of government programs: Public sector monies and legislative support are seldom bestowed without accompanying restrictions.[26] If the history of the HMO Act is repeated, more extensive governmental efforts to promote health care plans probably will be accompanied by new regulatory authority to restrict their organizational characteristics and modes of operation, again presumably in the consumer's interest.

There is a second reason to be cautious in the endorsement of increased governmental efforts to promote competitive health care plans as an indirect capacity-reduction strategy. The regulatory and administrative apparatus that would accompany government support could be used to limit the ability of health care plans to force hospitals to compete for their business. Faced with the choice of participating in a more competitive market or devoting effort to securing anticompetitive government rulings, hospitals may find that the latter option makes the greater economic sense. The potential for government effectively to foster the growth of competition may well rest with the ability of regulatory agencies to resist this type of pressure as it is applied by hospitals and other traditional providers.

A further consideration in government promotion of health care plans is the indirect nature of the connection between their development and reductions in excess hospital capacity. Initially, such plans could be expected to increase the number of empty hospital beds through reductions in unnecessary hospital utilization. This would not be an addition to excess capacity, but rather a conversion of existing excess capacity to a more obvious and less expensive form. Only after a potentially lengthy market adjustment period would reductions in hospital beds actually occur. However, in the short run, growth in the membership of health care plans might be perceived incorrectly by the public as contributing to the problem rather than aiding in its solution. This would make the encouragement of their development an unattractive strategy for politicians with necessarily short time horizons.

A Proposal for Public Sector Action

In summary, neither direct nor indirect approaches to hospital-capacity reduction promise a "quick fix" for a problem that has developed gradually over the past three decades. Direct approaches to capacity reduction have a strong surface attraction for politicians, since they give the electorate the impression that strong actions are being taken to stem rising hospital costs. However, we have argued that such approaches are likely to require uneconomically large amounts of resources to achieve even a moderate chance of success. Furthermore, since the direct elimination of hospital beds through public sector actions does not change the incentives that generated the excess capacity, a continuous long-run expenditure of public sector resources would be required just to maintain initial capacity reductions.

Indirect incentive-oriented strategies, although not without cost, seem to make greater economic sense. They have the crucial advantage of addressing the underlying cause of current excessive expenditures for hospital care—the lack of an appropriate incentive structure in the hospital industry. In particular, competition stimulated by health care plans would reward decision makers for developing and maintaining a long-term hospital capacity appropriate for their individual situations. Thus, the indirect approach offers some hope for a permanent solution. In contrast, direct attempts to reduce hospital capacity treat only one symptom of this lack of appropriate incentives, do not change the incentives themselves, and therefore offer little hope for a long-run solution.

Based on these considerations we propose that the public sector, and particularly HSAs, adopt a three-pronged approach to capacity reduction in the hospital industry.

(1) Promotion of Health Care Plans. Efforts should be made to alter capacity indirectly by pursuing policies that promise to change the incentives in the hospital industry and reward hospitals for eliminating their own excess capacities. These policies should focus primarily on promoting the development of health care plans. We believe that potentially effective government actions at the federal, state, and local levels include (a) the encouragement of business and labor to offer health care plans as health benefit options, (b) the active enforcement of antitrust laws where traditional providers attempt to limit the development and growth of health care plans, and (c) the modification of hospital-rate review and certificate-of-need programs to recognize the internal incentives of health care plans.

(2) Education of the Community. Because of the strength of interest groups which will resist attempts to reduce capacity through any method, broad-based community understanding and support is required if capacity is to be reduced. At the local level, HSAs should (a) publish comparisons of hospital costs per capita with those in other communities, calculations of the contribution of excess capacity to costs, and evidence of the lack of a demonstrated relationship between hospital capacity and community health; (b) establish goals for community per capita hospital expenditures; (c) establish goals with respect to hospital inputs (such as personnel) per capita, to help prevent the equating of hospital beds with capacity; and (d) emphasize the contribution that capacity reduction can make to achieving these goals.

(3) Establishment of a "Regulatory Threat." The threat of a "less desirable" regulatory alternative to voluntary cooperation may be necessary before hospitals will develop capacity-reduction plans or respond aggressively to competitive pressure. This regulation should be directed at altering the incentives of hospitals as much as possible, rather than

removing excess capacity directly. One regulatory alternative was discussed previously—the use of hospital-rate review programs to limit reimbursements for facilities with excess capacities. An even stronger step would be the imposition of a regulatory "lid" on community hospital expenditures, as an extension of the performance goals outlined above.[27] Such a lid would create strong incentives for hospitals to "police" each other. In conjunction with the expenditure lid, an attempt should be made to reward cost-effective hospitals by providing them with exemptions from selected existing regulations. This would strengthen the incentives of individual hospitals to alter their behavior. Because of the well-known problems inherent in regulatory proposals of all types, we expect that even a carefully constructed regulatory program would be more effective as a threat than as an implemented policy. It should be employed only as a last resort, since any public education or change of incentives accomplished by the first two public sector activities would increase the likelihood that subsequent regulatory action would be effective.

Having sketched what we believe to be the important components of a successful capacity-reduction strategy, it is appropriate to reiterate that hospital-capacity reduction is a means to an end, and not the end itself. The overall goal is the restraint of rapidly increasing hospital expenditures. Capacity reduction is only one of many approaches that might be taken to achieve this goal, and should be pursued only as long as it exhibits the greatest potential gain per dollar value of effort expended. In some areas, hospital-capacity reduction may meet this requirement. In other communities, it may not. The danger is that the present concern for capacity reduction will become an end in itself, diverting public and private sector resources from other, more appropriate means of containing expenditures and improving the health care system.

NOTES

1. Charles Schultze, *The Private Use of the Public Interest* (Washington, DC: Brookings, 1977), p. 65.

2. Walter McClure, *Reducing Excess Hospital Capacity,* NTIS HRP-0015199 [Department of Commerce] (Washington, DC: Government Printing Office, 1976), p. 5.

3. The higher estimate is found in *Controlling the Supply of Hospital Beds* (Washington, DC: National Academy of Sciences, 1976), pp. 15-16. The lower estimate is quoted by R. Bruce Andrews, Senior Vice President, American Medical International, Inc. in John K. Iglehart, "A Field Day for Goldilocks," *National Journal* (July 1978): 1060.

4. McClure, *Reducing Excess Hospital Capacity,* pp. 37-39.

5. Rockwell I. Schulz, and Jerry Rose, "Can Hospitals Be Expected to Control Costs?" *Inquiry* 10 (June 1975): 5.

6. The discussion in this section is a specific application of the economic literature on institutional change. See Terry L. Anderson, and P. J. Hill "Toward a General Theory of Institutional Change," *Frontiers of Economics* (1976), pp. 1-18: Victor P. Goldberg, "Institutional Change and the Quasi-Invisible Hand," *Journal of Law and Economics* 17 (October 1974): 461-492.

7. A detailed discussion of these two instruments and their relationship to other regulatory tools can be found in David A. Dittman and Jeffry A. Peters, "A Foundation for Health Care Regulation: PL 92-603 and PL 93-641," *Inquiry* (March 1977): 32-42.

8. The idea of appropriateness review for individual hospitals seems to have been delayed in its implementation indefinitely. Recent HEW rules (*Federal Register* 43, No 95, Tuesday, May 16, 1978) require only that institution-specific rules be phased in by HSAs as their resources allow.

9. Representative Paul Rogers has proposed a cost-control bill (H.R. 9717) that would allow for decertification of excess services designated through the appropriateness-review process.

10. Alain C. Enthoven, "Consumer-Choice Health Plan," *New England Journal of Medicine* 298 (1978): 655.

11. Bruce C. Vladeck, "Interest Group Representation and the HSAs: Health Planning and Political Theory," *American Journal of Public Health* 67 (January 1977): 26.

12. William G. Kopit, Edward J. Krill, and Karen F. Bonnie, "Hospital Decertification: Legitimate Regulation or Taking of Private Property?" *Utah Law Review* 179 (1978): 179-210.

13. Symond R. Gottlieb, "Reduction of Excess Hospital Capacity: A Suggested Strategy for Action," Greater Detroit Area Hospital Council, Inc., November 1977, p. 28.

14. Drew Altman, "The Politics of Health Care Regulation: The Case of the National Planning and Resources Development Act," *Journal of Health Politics, Policy and Law* 2 (Winter 1978): 560-580.

15. For example, Iowa has an occupancy rate of 72 percent and a bed supply of 5.5 per 1000 (1976). The national guidelines imply that relatively high per capita hospital costs should be observable in this area, but hospital costs are $170 per capita in Iowa versus the U.S. average of $187. Denver, with a 74 percent occupancy rate and 4.3 beds per 1000, should have lower per capita costs than Iowa according to a strict interpretation of the guidelines, yet it spends $200 per person in hospital care. Clearly the direct

relationship between bed supply, occupancy rates, and per capita costs implied in the guidelines is not universal. Consider a third community, Seattle-Tacoma, which already had a bed supply well under the guideline figure (3.3 per 1000 versus 4.0 per 1000). It has a low occupancy rate for its hospitals (71 percent) but also enjoys per capita hospital costs among the lowest in the nation ($158), primarily because of its low hospital use rate (860 versus 1239 patient days per thousand population for the U.S. average) and low hospital personnel rate (9.3 versus 11.5 per thousand population for the U.S. average). In short, these examples indicate that the guidelines are ill-suited to making community-by-community decisions with respect to appropriate hospital capacity. Their literal application in areas such as Seattle-Tacoma could actually increase community hospital costs. (Hospital data are taken from *Hospital Statistics,* 1977, while population data are from the *Statistical Abstract of the United States,* 1976).

16. Charles A. Frankenhoff, "The Planning Environment of Health Systems Agencies: A Strategy for Intervention," *Inquiry* 14 (1977): 218-219.

17. Schultze, *The Private Use,* p. 70.

18. McClure, *Reducing Excess Hospital Capacity,* p. 69.

19. Katherine G. Bauer, "Hospital Rate-Setting—This Way to Salvation?" *Milbank Memorial Fund Quarterly/Health and Society* 55 (Winter 1977): 49.

20. Another method for restructuring the incentives in the market for hospital services is described by Joseph P. Newhouse, and V. Taylor "How Shall We Pay for Hospital Care?" *The Public Interest* 23 (Spring 1971): 78-92.

21. Walter McClure, "On Broadening the Definition and Removing Regulatory Barriers to a Competitive Health Care System," *Journal of Health Politics, Policy and Law* 3 (Fall 1978): 303-327.

22. For a detailed description of the Twin Cities market, see Jon B. Christianson, and Walter McClure, "Competition in the Delivery of Medical Care," *New England Journal of Medicine* 301 (October 11, 1979): 812-818.

23. The procedures used to project the impact of HMO enrollment growth on the use of hospital beds in the Twin Cities under various assumptions are described in detail in Jon B.Christianson, and Walter McClure, *Private and Public Approaches to Excess Hospital Capacity and Health Care Expenditures,* (Excelsior, MN: Interstudy, 1978).

24. Paul Starr, "The Undelivered Health Care System," *The Public Interest* 42 (Winter 1976): 76.

25. Ibid., p. 77.

26. Schultze, *The Private Use, pp. 71-72.*

27. The "Rochester Project" provides an interesting model in this regard and is summarized by Andrew A. Sorenson and Ernest W. Saward, "An Alternative Approach to Hospital Cost Control: The Rochester Project," *Public Health Reports* 93 (July-August 1978): 311-368.

Chapter 7

Long-Term Care Standards

Enforcement and Compliance

The Medicaid and Medicare programs have dramatically expanded government's role as a financier of medical care and have increased public concern with the nature of the care purchased. Regulatory bodies have found it extremely difficult to assess the relative quality of medical care and, as a consequence, have assumed a strong relationship exists between the nature of inputs in the production of medical care and its quality. This assumption has been used to support restrictions on the way medical services must be produced to qualify for governmental reimbursement. The following discussion examines restrictions placed on the providers of long-term care. The development of regulation in this industry is reviewed in the context of competing models of regulatory behavior. The discussion rejects simplistic views of the motivations of regulators as inconsistent with the historical evidence and the enforcement incentives facing individual inspectors. Small

Authors' Note: *From Jon B. Christianson, "Long-Term Care Standards: Enforcement and Compliance,"* Journal of Health Politics, Policy and Law, *Vol. 4, No. 3 (Fall 1979), pp. 414-434. Copyright© 1979 by the Department of Health Administration, Duke University. Reprinted by permission. The research upon which this chapter is based was performed pursuant to grant APR75-16570 with the National Science Foundation. The author thanks Theodore R. Marmor and Oscar R. Burt for their comments.*

sample data concerning the effect of regulation on provider incomes and the relationship between reported compliance with standards and provider operating costs are examined. They prove consistent with a theory of regulatory behavior based on the self-interest of the participating parties. The chapter concludes by addressing proposals for reforming the provision of long-term care with respect to their probable impacts on the enforcement of standards.

The Development of Long-Term Care Standards

Background

Expenditures on long-term care have increased dramatically during the past fifteen years, as shown in Table 7.1. This increase is a combined result of inflation, population growth, increased per capita utilization because of third-party payment, and modifications in the content of the long-term care product due to technological change and change ordered through regulation. The influence of population growth can be removed from the data by deflating aggregate expenditures by number of recipients; similarly, price indices can be used to convert actual expenditures to "real" dollars. Yet, even when deflated for population growth and inflation, yearly real per capita expenditure on long-term care remains impressive: at least a 108 percent increase between 1967 and 1975 and an average annual growth rate of 10.6 percent.

During this period of rapid expenditure growth, and particularly growth in the proportion of expenditures deriving from the public sector (see Table 7.1), there was increasing concern about the quality of care provided in nursing homes. This concern resulted in more active regulation of providers.[1] Provider licensing programs, which existed in most states prior to Medicaid and Medicare, were supplemented by a more stringent and uniform set of federal input-oriented regulations. Compliance with these regulations, as judged by state enforcement agencies, became necessary for certification as an

TABLE 7.1 Expenditures on Long-Term Care[a]

Fiscal Year	*Expenditures (in millions)* Total	Private	Public	*Percentage Distribution* Private	Public	*Per Capita Expenditure*	*Real Per Capita Expenditure[b] (1967 = 1000)* Medical Care	Hospital Semi-private Room
1960	480	NA	NA	NA	NA	2.63	3.32	4.59
1965	1271	NA	NA	NA	NA	6.46	7.22	8.51
1966	1407	NA	NA	NA	NA	7.07	7.56	8.47
1967	1751	844	907	48.2	51.8	8.70	8.70	8.70
1968	2360	894	1466	37.9	62.1	11.60	10.93	10.21
1969	3057	1354	1703	44.3	55.7	14.89	13.11	11.56
1970	3818	2145	1673	56.2	43.8	18.40	15.26	12.65
1971	4890	2919	1971	59.7	40.3	23.34	18.18	14.31
1972	5860	3395	2465	57.9	42.1	27.70	20.91	15.93
1973	6650	3477	3173	52.3	47.7	31.19	22.65	17.13
1974	7450	3574	3876	48.0	52.0	34.69	23.05	17.22
1975	9000	3799	5201	42.2	57.8	41.55	24.91	18.06

a. Health, United States, 1975. DHEW (HRA) 76-1232: 69, 1976; Mueller, M. S., and Gibson, R.M.: National Health Expenditures. Fiscal Year 1975. Social Security Bulletin, February 3, 1976.

b. Per capita expenditures based on the total United States population are adjusted by the medical care price index and the price index for a hospital semi-private room. Actual expenditures per capita in year n are multiplied by the ratio of the price index in base year (1967) to the price index in year n. Although nursing home services are not included when computing the medical care price index, this index does reflect price pressure in the medical care market in general. Inputs used in providing a hospital semi-private room are similar in many cases to those used in providing long-term care in a nursing home. Therefore there should be some correlation between prices in these two settings.

extended care facility (Medicare) or a skilled nursing home (Medicaid) and consequently for the receipt of federal reimbursement funds. The relationship between regulatory compliance (particularly in skilled nursing homes) and federal reimbursement quickly became controversial. Officials in the Department of Health, Education, and Welfare (DHEW) were accused of lowering standards, granting unnecessary waivers, postponing deadlines, and, as a result, subverting the intent of the regulatory legislation.[2] State inspectors were accused of being ill-trained and poorly supervised in the performance of their duties. An internal audit conducted by DHEW seemed to support these contentions; it revealed a minimum of 227 substandard nursing homes containing 6453 beds receiving Medicaid funds during 1969 in California alone.[3] Further evidence was supplied in a report issued by the U.S. Senate's Committee on Finance in 1970. Of 4776 facilities certified as extended care facilities in 1969, only 1374 were judged to be in full compliance with certification requirements.[4]

Congress attempted to upgrade this record of regulatory performance through a series of amendments to the Social Security Act (1972) directed in part at increasing the authority of government agencies in dealing with violators. These amendments also required a unification of Medicare and Medicaid standards pertaining to long-term care. In ordering the development of uniform standards by DHEW, Congress apparently intended that the new regulations reflect the more stringent requirements of the Medicare program. However, in implementing this directive DHEW interpreted the intent of Congress as defining a lowest acceptable level of care.[5] Since the 1972 amendments there have been numerous other initiatives directed at increased government control of long-term care providers and the development of more effective enforcement mechanisms. It is the implementation of, and compliance with, these standards that this chapter seeks to understand.

Models of Regulatory Behavior

The historical development of long-term care regulation seems to have been cyclical in nature—disappointing provider performance resulting in new, "tougher" regulations, consequent increased expectations, and further disillusionment when these expectations were not fulfilled. If this cycle is to be altered in the future, the motives of long-term care regulators must be understood.

There are two prominent approaches to explaining regulatory behavior.[6] The more traditional approach emphasizes the need to protect consumers from the actions of producers. According to this view, producers often dominate consumers because their market power permits charging "inappropriately" high prices and thus accumulating "inappropriately" large profits. This is accomplished through control over the formation of potential competitors or through the provision of an inferior product. Therefore the purpose of the regulatory system is to protect consumers by placing constraints on the market power of producers. This is termed the "public interest" concept of regulation.

The "self-interest" theory of regulatory behavior is the antithesis of the public interest approach. It argues that existing firms extract benefits from regulations through "capture" of the regulatory body. Once "captured," the regulators can be used to fix prices, limit the entry of new firms, restrict the development of substitute products, and in general promote policies that increase profits in the regulated industry.[7]

These two approaches lead to quite different conclusions when applied to long-term care regulations and their growth. The public interest theory would portray input regulations as attempts to protect the consumer—the nursing home resident—from poorly trained personnel, unsafe physical surroundings, and inappropriate treatments. A very important by-product is the assurance that the public sector is purchasing services of some acceptable value for its expenditure of tax dollars. The body of regulations then grew in response to attempts by providers to supply low-quality care (assuming this quality can be measured) and to increases in the proportion of the long-term care bill paid by government. The public statements of consumer groups and legislators reflect this view of the long-term care regulatory process, but overlook a consequence of these regulations. In effect, long-term care standards limit the range of competitors faced by existing firms. They restrict the nature of the product being sold and the choice of providers available to Medicaid and Medicare eligibles. Therefore one might expect that existing firms which meet new standards would support their strict definition and enforcement. This provides one explanation for the lobbying for more stringent standards carried out by the nonprofit segment of the industry,[8] an effort at odds with the public interest view of regulatory behavior.

The self-interest theory would predict this type of behavior by existing long-term care firms, since it is in their interest to limit competition. It also would predict efforts on the part of provider groups to increase reimbursement levels. Providers cite increases in the cost of care induced by regulations to support their arguments for higher Medicaid and Medicare payments. There is some prima facie evidence of success in these efforts. The Senate Subcommittee on Long-Term Care found that corporate nursing homes enjoyed increases of 122.6 percent in total assets, 149.5 percent in gross revenues, and 116 percent in average net income during the period from 1969 to 1972. The subcommittee further suggests that these results are consistent with the experience of individual operators as well.[9] While impressive, these data do not necessarily imply that the regulatory body has been captured. The capture theory implies that the profits of Medicaid and Medicare providers would be larger than the profits of providers specializing in private patients. Therefore there would be considerable incentive to secure patients eligible for federal reimbursement. Recent evidence does not support this prediction.[10] In many states a substantial number of nursing homes have voluntarily relinquished their Medicaid and Medicare certification. One has a difficult time reconciling this behavior with regulatory agencies that have been captured by long-term care providers and used for their benefit.

Conflicting Interests in Regulation

The public interest and self-interest theories draw attention to different aspects of the regulation of long-term care, but neither is consistent with the broad patterns of regulatory policy and provider response. A theory containing elements of both ought to explain more successfully the development and enforcement of long-term care regulations. Such an approach accepts the public interest notion that regulatory bodies attempt to serve the public, not the regulated firm, but acknowledges that they are confronted with severe difficulties in achieving this objective. The information upon which regulators base their actions is likely to be uncertain and biased. Since the public interest cannot be precisely defined, they must balance pressures from numerous groups with conflicting interests and abilities to press these interests. The self-interest of providers represents only one factor they must consider. When conducting their "balancing act," Noll has suggested that regulators have three general goals:[11]

(1) minimizing the extent to which their decisions are overturned through court actions;
(2) securing a favorable response from legislators to agency decisions; and
(3) promoting satisfactory performance on the part of the regulated industry.

Regulatory agencies face conflicting demands that make any determination of the public interest controversial and unstable. There is a clear intent expressed by legislators at the federal level to improve patient conditions through more demanding regulation of inputs. However, long-term care firms have argued that this would add to costs without corresponding increases in reimbursement, making participation in Medicaid and Medicare programs financially unattractive. This could result in an insufficient supply of beds for Medicaid and Medicare eligibles.

These conflicting pressures place DHEW in a quandry. Legislative approval requires the support of stricter standards and stronger enforcement efforts, but risks an industry performance failure. The DHEW interpretation of legislative intent concerning uniform Medicare and Medicaid standards and its authorization of federal reimbursement payments to facilities not in compliance with regulations (see above) demonstrates that it has been sensitive to industry arguments. Passage of the 1972 amendments to the Social Security Act (also referred to in previous discussion) is evidence of legislative displeasure with DHEW's strategy. DHEW's response to these conflicting pressures is predictable when one considers the relative strengths and incentives of the interested parties.[12] The immediate costs of restrictive regulations (assuming that they are only imperfectly passed on in the form of higher reimbursement rates) are concentrated on long-term care providers. Therefore, many providers, particularly those with profit incentives, have a strong motivation to oppose these restrictions. Their interest in long-term care regulation will lead them to maintain a continuous, well-supported effort to press their views. Providers are likely to be complemented in these efforts by other governmental departments attempting to maintain or increase their own shares of the budget. It is in the interest of these departments to oppose regulations that will increase the program costs and budget shares of Medicaid and Medicare.[13]

State agencies dealing with the regulation of long-term care also face conflicting interests in their performance. They are responsible for developing reimbursement structures and financing a portion of the Medicaid long-term care bill from state funds. They also have the responsibility for inspection of providers and certification of compliance with federal and other standards. Federal regulations require states to develop reimbursement structures that enlist participation by enough providers so that services are available to Medicaid eligibles to the same extent that they are available to the general population.[14]

However, competition from other state agencies and, in certain instances, legislative displeasure with rising Medicaid state budget shares have led some states to limit reimbursement rates and reduce covered services. The defection of providers from the Medicaid program (which accompanied these decisions) has resulted in litigation pending against at least one state government.[15]

Apparently the Medicaid coverage and reimbursement levels advocated by consumer groups and providers would not be attractive to state regulators, since they are unlikely to be approved by legislatures. However, in supporting alternative plans which fail to elicit provider participation, regulatory agencies risk having their policies overturned through court action. It is difficult to predict the response of state regulatory agencies to this conflict, since there are concentrated and continuing interests (state agencies versus providers) representing both viewpoints.

The conflicting goals of providers, citizen groups and their legislative representatives, and governmental agencies make it necessary for regulatory policymakers in long-term care to pursue multiple objectives. These regulatory objectives are weighted by the relative abilities of the various groups in influencing the decision-making process.[16] The public interest view of regulatory policy abstracts from the difficulty of determining which decisions are in the public interest when legitimate goals are in conflict. The self-interest approach proposes a one-dimensional objective—the welfare of the regulated firm—which also suffers from its lack of realism. The "political marketplace" view of regulation provides a superior explanation of the long-term care regulatory process because it acknowledges the complicated demands faced by the regulator.

Enforcement

Inherent in any regulatory enforcement process are the incentives that define the relationship between the inspector and the regulated firm. Inspectors of long-term care facilities are in frequent contact with providers and thus become familiar with, and very probably sympathetic to, their difficulties in complying with standards. The personal incentives of inspectors are to minimize job-related conflict situations and unpleasantness by practicing lenient enforcement, or negotiation rather than prosecution, as long as the costs of acting in this manner are small.[17] This does not imply that inspectors are corrupt or incompetent. It does suggest that they will behave normally with respect to employment incentives.

This conclusion would require modification if the interests of other parties to the regulatory process favored strict enforcement of standards and if these parties had the means and incentive to press their interests on inspectors. Then the cost to inspectors of minimizing job conflict would increase, and stricter enforcement of standards would result. However, one could argue plausibly that the reverse is true; often the interests of other groups also favor lenient enforcement. For instance, the minimization of job conflict is also a relevant objective for supervisors in the inspection process. They do not wish to deal with continual complaints from providers concerning "callous" enforcement of "unreasonable" standards. Therefore they cannot be expected to argue for stricter enforcement on their own initiative. The interests of state legislators and other state government departments, as already argued, will not provide consistent pressures for enforcement. These parties will probably evaluate the social costs and benefits of enforcement incorrectly. The costs of enforcement, both in terms of direct state expenditures and increased risk of under provision of the regulated good, are obvious and immediate. Stricter enforcement of standards supposedly improves the quality of care, but this benefit is difficult to assess. It also accrues by relatively small amounts over a long period of time and is spread over a large number of recipients. Furthermore, the connection between legislative efforts and subsequent improvements in quality of care may be hard for the politician to establish. All of these factors make the strict enforcement of long-term care standards a relatively unattractive issue to pursue for the vote-conscious politician with an understandably limited time horizon. For these same reasons, enforcement pressures are not likely to derive from politicians and agencies at the federal level.

The task of monitoring the enforcement process therefore rests with citizen groups interested in improving the quality of care. They can be influential when responding to highly visible results of ineffective enforcement, such as fire, Medicaid kickback schemes, or the misuse of drugs. In these cases, it may be possible to mobilize legislative support for reform. However, as often has been noted, voluntary public interest groups cannot be expected to be effective as monitors of the day-to-day regulatory process. The benefits of such actions are simply too diffuse relative to the costs of monitoring. Consequently public interest in the regulatory problems of long-term care will tend to be sporadic, triggered by flagrant abuses or journalistic expose.

In addition to the incentives deriving from the political marketplace for regulation, the existing institutional framework discourages strong enforcement efforts by inspectors. The fragmented assignment of responsibility among governmental bodies, the length of time involved in the enforcement process, and the lack of alternative penalties for violators all have contributed to the ineffectiveness of the enforcement process.[18] Inspection of long-term care facilities is carried out by state health departments. (There may be additional fire-safety and building inspections conducted by local governments.) If a violation is uncovered in the first inspection, the facility is given a specific time period in which to correct the deficiency or submit a plan detailing the manner in which the deficiency will be corrected. This is followed by a second inspection and possibily a second notice to the facility requesting that the deficiency be corrected. If the notice is ignored or the deficiency is not adequately corrected in the opinion of the inspector, prosecution of the violator can be recommended. The prosecutor, who works for a different government agency, may have a heavy caseload and therefore not act on the recommendation of the inspector. A conviction may result in the payment of a minimal fine at one extreme or the much more serious loss of certification and federal monies. The lack of an appropriate range of penalties probably increases the likelihood that a conviction will cost the facility very little and therefore have little deterrent value.

Marginal Benefits and Costs

The political marketplace for long-term care standards and the enforcement procedures that have developed as a consequence do not support a simplistic view of the long-term care regulatory process. The failure of DHEW and state agencies to pursue a more active enforcement policy does not necessarily imply that they have been "captured" by the industry; nor does it imply a technical inability on their part to perform this task. Instead, it suggests that incomplete enforcement is a rational and entirely understandable decision given the performance objectives of regulatory agencies and individual inspectors. It arguably contributes to the availability of long-term beds and therefore to the ability of the industry to meet the demand for its services, an important indicator of successful performance for federal and state regulators. For the participating agencies there is an optimal level of enforcement of regulations:[19] They can be expected to pursue their enforcement duties only to the point where the marginal costs (measured in terms of the political consequences of restricted supply and increased program costs as well as the personal discomfort of increased job conflict) equal the marginal benefits (derived from the political goodwill of citizen groups and legislators representing their interests). Thus, one should expect to observe less than complete enforcement of, and compliance with, long-term care standards, since this is a potentially optimal strategy for the regulatory agencies involved.

Empirical Evidence

The preceding discussion raises several issues concerning the impact of long-term care regulations in a setting characterized by uncertain and incomplete compliance. In this section two hypotheses are investigated further. The first hypothesis examines the assertion by providers that more restrictive input requirements reduce profits. The second considers the possibility that the existing inspection process is an unreliable indicator of firm performance in complying with regulations. The empirical analysis is based on data from actual firm experience. This is preferable to simulation analysis grounded on assumptions of complete regulatory compliance and fixed technologies. The previous discussion suggests that such simulations overestimate regulatory costs to the firm.

Data

Data are required on long-term care provider expenses, operating income, operating characteristics, and compliance with existing regulations. The State of Montana Department of Social Rehabilitation Services collects data in the first three categories through reports filed annually by facilities receiving Medicaid reimbursements. Of the approximately eighty facilities participating in these programs in 1974, forty-five authorized access to their reports under the assurance of anonymity. The reports provide data on ownership, licensure of beds in different classifications, occupancy, number of beds, expenses in various administrative categories, and income. Some facilities are combination hospital/nursing homes, and their data proved to be unusable since they did not isolate expenses incurred solely by nursing home beds. Eliminating these facilities and providers for which data are missing or reporting procedures suspect reduces the sample size to thirty. The final sample

TABLE 7.2 Facility Characteristics

Variable	*Mean Value*
Ownership (0 = nonprofit; 1 = for-profit)	.42
Number of beds	59.00
Proportion of beds licensed for skilled nursing care	.59
Proportion of beds licensed for intermediate care A	.32
Total operating expense per patient day	16.01
Total operating income per patient day	15.16
Number of violations	22.35

contains a disproportionate number of nonprofit firms partially because all publicly owned facilities are required to disclose their reports.[20] Summary data on the sample are provided in Table 7.2.

Until 1972, data on compliance with federal standards were difficult to obtain. In that year, Congress adopted legislation requiring DHEW to make available to the public information on regulatory violations as collected by state inspectors. By 1974, summaries of these reports were available for public inspection at Social Security offices. Data on violations were abstracted from summaries filed on participating Medicaid long-term are facilities in Montana during 1974 and early 1975.

Each violation recorded in the summaries was placed into one of fourteen general categories based on the inspector's worksheet. A judgmental distinction was made between violations which referred to the incorrect completion of a form required by Medicaid/Medicare for documentation purposes, and more substantive deficiencies, such as inadequate physical plant, inappropriate staffing, omission of required procedures in the delivery of care, or the total absence of necessary utilization-review plans or consultation agreements. The results of this categorization process are presented in Table 7.3.

Twenty-five percent of the reported deficiencies pertained to the physical environment of the long-term care facility. They were largely violations in the controversial "life-safety" code, such as inadequate sprinkler systems, nonaccommoda-

TABLE 7.3 Classification of Violations

Violations	Substantive		Paperwork		Combined		
	Total	*Average*	*Total*	*Average*	*Total*	*Average*	*Percentage*
Governing body and management	227	2.8	97	1.2	324	4.1	17.2
Medical direction and physician services	62	.8	36	.5	98	1.2	5.2
Nursing services	58	.8	30	.4	88	1.1	4.7
Dietetic services	83	.9	23	.3	106	1.3	5.6
Rehabilitative and radiological services	48	.6	22	.3	70	.9	3.7
Dental services	39	.5	10	.1	49	.6	2.6
Social services and patient activities	110	1.4	50	.6	160	2.0	8.5
Medical records	99	1.2	13	.2	112	1.4	6.0
Transfer agreement	7	.1	3	.04	10	.1	.5
Physical environment	457	5.7	17	.2	474	.59	25.2
Infection Control	62	.8	29	.4	91	1.1	4.8
Disaster preparedness	78	1.0	15	.2	93	1.2	4.9
Utilization review	14	.2	4	.05	18	.2	1.0
Pharmaceutical services	153	1.9	36	.5	189	2.4	10.0
Total	1497	18.7	385	4.8	1882	23.5	100.0

tion of facilities to wheelchairs, doors and corridors of inappropriate sizes, and the absence of emergency warning systems for the blind and deaf. Violations classified under "governing body and management," the second largest category in terms of number of deficiencies, concerned the lack of required written plans or procedures for various aspects of a facility's operation. Typical in this regard were inadequate, outdated, or nonexistent plans for capital expenditure, continuing education of personnel, safeguarding of patient personal possessions, obtaining blood for transfusions, patient discharge, and development of a patient bill of rights.

These data on compliance were then combined with the data on characteristics, expenses, and income for the thirty facilities. The compliance performance in the sample corresponded closely with the data presented for all eighty facilities in Table 7.3. The mean number of violations for all facilities was 23.5, while the same mean for the sample of thirty was 22.4.

Bed Certification

There are four levels of certification for long-term care beds in Montana: skilled nursing care, intermediate A, intermediate B, and boarding. The most stringent standards are applied to beds certified as skilled nursing care beds, with standards for the other three classifications becoming progressively more lenient. Stricter standards require the more intensive use of labor and other inputs in the provision of care. Therefore, if a high proportion of beds in a given facility are licensed as skilled nursing care or intermediate A, one would expect relatively high expenses for patient care in that facility. To test this hypothesis, a regression equation was estimated with operating expenses per patient day as the dependent variable and ownership (profit or nonprofit), number of beds, number of beds squared, proportion of total beds licensed as skilled nursing care, proportion of total beds licensed as intermediate A, and recorded violations as explanatory variables. The use of variables for ownership and bed size is common to nursing home cost analysis. Occupancy rates, another commonly used variable, were not included in the analysis since they were extremely high in the sample and exhibited little variation. Because of data limitations no attempt was made to control for the medical condition of patients. One would expect a high correlation between the proportion of certified skilled nursing beds in a facility and the seriousness of the medical condition of its residents. Finally, preliminary analysis showed no relationship between expenses and location of the facility in a small community, so this variable was also omitted.

Results of the analysis of expenses are given in Table 7.4. The signs of the estimated coefficients for the explantory variables in the operating expense equation are as hypothesized. For profit facilities can be expected to have operating expenses per patient day that are $2.40 less than those of their nonprofit counterparts. The coefficients on the variables relating to number of beds indicate that expenses per patient day decrease as facility size increases over the range of the data. Theoretically, the total number of regulatory violations should bear an inverse relationship to expenses, a lower number of violations indicating a greater degree of regulatory compliance and hence higher costs per patient day. The sign of the estimated coefficient supports this hypothesis; however, the magnitude of the estimate is very small and its significance extremely low.

Of primary interest are the estimated coefficients for the bed certification variables. Both coefficients are statistically significant and indicate that the proportion of beds certified under the more stringent regulatory requirements has a positive effect on costs. The exact interpretation of these estimates is not obvious and therefore deserves some explanation. Assume that a facility of one hundred beds has sixty certified for skilled nursing care, twenty for care at the intermediate A level, and twenty for intermediate B care. Its costs per patient day would average $.82 greater than a one-hundred-bed facility with fifty skilled nursing, twenty intermediate A, and thirty intermediate B beds; or $.34 greater (.822-.477) than a facility with fifty

TABLE 7.4 Regression Results: Income and Expenses (N = 30; standard deviations in parentheses)

	Ownership[a]	*Bed Size*	*Bed Size Squared*	*Proportion of Beds Licensed Skilled Nursing Care*	*Proportion of Beds Licensed Intermediate A*	*Total Number of Violations*	*Intercept*	R^2	*F-Test*
Operating Income per patient day	.57	−.066**	.00034**	7.03***	3.78*	−.0016	11.66	.41	2.62**
	(1.09)	(.041**)	(.00017)	(2.29)	(2.40)	(.053)			
Operating Expense per patient day	−2.25***	−.083**	.00041**	8.22***	4.77**	−.004	13.49	.51	3.98***
	(1.16)	(.044)	(.00018)	(2.46)	(2.57)	(.057)			

*statistically significant 90% confidence level
**statistically significant 95% confidence level
***statistically significant 99% confidence level
a. 1 = for-profit; 0 = nonprofit

skilled nursing, thirty intermediate A, and twenty intermediate B beds.

These cost differences cannot be attributed entirely to regulation through bed certification. In fact, bed certification may have formalized an intuitively obvious proposition—patients receive different levels of care dependent on their medical conditions. In order to measure the addition to costs due to the certification procedure, one might estimate these costs for facilities before and after they were certified while holding the distribution of patients by medical condition constant. However, this would ignore other costs associated with regulation. For instance, a facility may find itself with more certified skilled nursing care beds than it has patients requiring care at this level. If this results in the placement of patients requiring lower levels of treatment into skilled nursing beds, resources devoted to patient care will be greater than necessary. This is a more subtle, and certainly more difficult to quantify, "cost of regulation."

Although the effect of bed certification on costs is an interesting issue in itself, it is perhaps less controversial than the relationship between bed certification and net operating income. To investigate this relationship, a regression equation was estimated with the same set of explanatory factors (as in the expense equation) but with operating income as the dependent variable. The results are presented in Table 7.4. Both the nonprofit and for-profit firms have incentives to maximize operating income per patient day, but these incentives differ in origin and probably in importance. The for-profit firm views income maximization as essential for profit maximization. The administrator of a nonprofit facility has a somewhat weaker incentive, viewing income maximization as a means of increasing the funds under his or her control. The estimated ownership coefficient is statistically insignificant, indicating that variation in income cannot be explained on the basis of the relative strength of these incentives.

To the extent that violations are publicized, one would expect them to be a negative factor in the consumer's choice of facility. In order to attract residents, facilities with poor violation records could be expected to lower charges with a resulting lower operating income per patient day. The sign of the coefficient supports this hypothesis but the estimate is statistically insignificant. This no doubt reflects demand pressures and the lack of publicity given to long-term care regulatory compliance.[21]

The coefficients on the certification variables are significant and demonstrate that income increases as the proportion of beds in the more stringently regulated categories increases. This, of course, is to be expected, since reimbursement levels in these categories are higher. Of primary interest, however, is the relationship between these marginal effects on income and the similar effects on expenses as the proportion of skilled nursing and intermediate A beds increases. The estimates indicate that higher proportions of beds in the skilled nursing and intermediate A categories result in larger marginal additions to cost than to income. However, this result is not statistically significant. On the basis of the statistical evidence one cannot reject the hypothesis that an increased proportion of total beds in the more stringently regulated categories would have an equal effect on expenses and income. That is, one cannot conclude that facilities are affected adversely in terms of net income by submitting to more intensive regulation.

Compliance Performance

If regulatory standards are costly to comply with, then those long-term care firms with the fewest violations should experience the greatest expenses, ceteris paribus.[22] This assumes that compliance as reported through the enforcement process accurately reflects actual firm performance. If the incentives outlined above are correct, it seems more likely that there would be no empirical relationship between reported compliance with regulations and firm costs. This result would support our analysis of the enforcement process in long-term care but would not be conclusive. Therefore, other explanations for the lack of a statistically significant relationship between these two variables also must be investigated.

In the estimated expense equation in Table 7.4, total violations per facility is not a significant explanatory variable for total operating expenses per patient day. However, it is possible that the level of aggregation for both expenses and violations disguised relationships that exist at a more disaggregate level. In order to examine this possibility, regression equations were estimated for expense categories which could be matched with similar categories of regulatory deficiencies as described in Table 7.2. For instance, administrative expenses per patient day (which included salaries for administrative and clerical employees) were regressed against the original set of explanatory variables and the number of "paper" violations, with the expectation that a good performance in meeting the clerical requirements of Medicaid/Medicare would be reflected in higher expenditures in this category. For the remainder of the expense categories, "substantive," as opposed to "paper," violations were used as explanatory variables, since these "substantive" violations were most likely to be related to costs and therefore to be successful in explaining variations in costs.

The regression results (Table 7.5) show a mixed performance in terms of statistical significance for the independent variables with the exception of the violation variables. The significance of these variables is uniformly low, with an average confidence level of 60 percent. This performance was probably not related to the presence of multicollinearity among the independent variables; no more than 35 percent of the variation in any violation variable can be explained by a regression on the remaining explanatory variables. Nor is it the result of a lack of variation in reported compliance; total violations ranged from ten to forty-nine, with comparable variation observed in the violations for the disaggregated expense categories.

It could be argued that ordinary least squares regression techniques are not appropriate for estimation of the group of

TABLE 7.5 Regression Results: Expenses and Regulatory Compliance (ordinary least squares, N = 30; standard deviations in parentheses)

	Ownership[a]	*Bed Size*	*Bed Size Squared*	*Proportion of Beds Licensed Skilled Nursing Care*	*Proportion of Beds Licensed Intermediate A*	*Total Number of Violations*	*Intercept*	R^2	*F-Test*
Administrative	1.034***	−.011	.00004	.433	−.438	−.015	1.922	.34	1.99
	(.378)	(.0145)	(.00006)	(.85)	(.91)	(.059)			
Dietary	−.628***	−.012*	.00004	1.758***	1.442***	−.069	2.315	.54	4.42***
	(.236)	(.0087)	(.000036)	(.48)	(.50)	(.08)			
Nursing service	−1.735***	−.032*	.00016**	2.602***	1.44	−.38	6.345	.57	4.99***
	(.61)	(.02)	(.00008)	(1.15)	(1.17)	(.41)			
Service (lab, x-ray, therapy)	−.009	−.001	.000013***	.066	.061	.021	−.007		
	(.038)	(.0014)	(.000006)	(.079)	(.08)	(.035)		.51	3.93***
Pharmacy	.03	−.0023	.00003***	.124	.053	.0024	−.020	.65	7.1***
	(.057)	(.002)	(.000009)	(.123)	(.12)	(.021)			
Maintenance	−.50**	.00096	−.0000017	.145	−.075	−.009	.740	.20	.99
	(.237)	(.009)	(.000036)	(.49)	(.5)	(.024)			

*statistically significant at 90% confidence level
**statistically significant at 95% confidence level
***statistically significant at 99% confidence level
a. 1 = for-profit; 0 = nonprofit

expense relations. In particular, one might expect that the expense equations are related through their error terms. A random influence causing a positive disturbance in one expense category for a given facility would quite likely cause disturbances in the same direction for the remaining expense classifications. If this is the case, the efficiency of the ordinary least squares technique is questionable. More precise estimates of the coefficients on the violations variables (and possibly higher levels of significance) might be obtained by employing a technique that takes into account the disturbance simultaneity. There is both theoretical and experimental evidence indicating that a two-stage Aitken estimator produces smaller variances under these conditions than does ordinary least squares even when sample size is small.[23] However, the use of this estimator resulted in almost no increase in the significance of the violation variables.

The insignificance of the violation variables could suggest that there is slack in the use of existing resources in some long-term care firms. If employees are not being fully utilized, then they can be devoted to regulatory compliance activities without increasing costs per patient day. This would make any empirical relationship between compliance and costs unlikely. Theoretically, since their incentives to minimize costs are weaker, nonprofit firms are more likely to enjoy this "slack" than their for-profit counterparts. Therefore, a change in costs corresponding to a change in compliance would vary with ownership status if the slack explanation were correct. To test this hypothesis an interaction term (defined as the product of the ownership and violation variables) was introduced in the regression equations of Tables 7.4 and 7.5. The estimated coefficients for these interaction variables were insignificant, providing no support for the slack hypothesis.

The discretion given to individual inspectors, the incentives for inspectors to be lenient, and the use of different inspectors with varying personal standards all suggest that reported violations have questionable informational content. This might explain their lack of significance in the estimated model.

However, the observed lack of statistical significance is merely consistent with this explanation, and does not conclusively support it. There may be other as yet unexplored, explantions for the empirical results which are equally plausible.

Reforming the Regulatory Process

The continued growth of public expenditures on long-term care and the difficulties of regulating providers have led to numerous reform proposals for this industry. These proposals have ranged from limited attempts to change the inspection process to relatively major suggestions for industry reorganization. Most of these proposals ignore the fundamental imbalance in the political marketplace for long-term care regulation and reimbursement.

The 1974 Long-Term Care Facility Improvement Campaign funded improved training programs for inspectors as a means of tightening the enforcement of standards. The development of alternatives to decertification as punishment for noncompliance is an institutional reform with much the same objective. While training programs may improve the competence of inspectors in recognizing deficiencies, they do not alter incentives for lenient enforcement. The existence of alternative models for punishing providers should result in the prosecution of more reported violations, but will not necessarily result in stronger efforts to uncover regulatory deficiencies. Neither reform addresses the imbalances in the political marketplace which shape the incentives of long-term care regulators.

A recent reform effort has been directed at replacing input-oriented regulations with evaluation of output.[24] If a satisfactory method for evaluating quality of care can be developed, this would make the somewhat suspect assumption that increased inputs result in improved care no longer necessary. Reimbursement could be linked with the provision of an acceptable quality of care rather than the use of a specified set of inputs. Although this would shift the attention of the regulatory process to a more appropriate issue, the interests and relative strengths of the participants would be changed very little. Indeed, depending on the measurement instrument developed, the regulator may find that nonenforcement has become more difficult to detect.

Although the reimbursement of providers for services and their compliance with regulations are closely related, proposals for reform of the reimbursement process usually do not address regulatory enforcement issues. In fact, Ruchlin, Levey, and Muller state that "the correction of facility deficiencies requires a concentrated effort on the part of regulatory agencies. It is not a problem susceptible to direct amelioration by the reimbursement process, nor should it be."[25] On the basis of this chapter, one might argue that such a "concentrated effort" will not be soon forthcoming.

Shulman and Galanter have proposed a reform that theoretically does address the imbalance of interests in the marketplace for long-term care. They have suggested that the nursing home industry be reorganized "with capital facilities owned by the government, but with management conducted through a system of competitive contracts with the private sector."[26] This system, they argue, would create a new set of participants in the regulatory process with strong incentives to uncover and report violations of standards. "Instead of relying only on patients and inspectors for word of contract violations, government would now also have available the resources of competitors for the contract. Firms anxious to succeed in the nursing home management business would have strong financial incentives to report their competitors' failings through the public-review/contract-award process."[27] In practice, the effectiveness of this reform in altering the existing balance of regulatory interests depends crucially on the nature of the contract that is adopted. Given the existing interests and resources of those parties who would oppose the plan, it is doubtful that the ideal contract proposed by Shulman and Galanter would survive the machinations of legislators and bureaucrats.[28] Nevertheless, their reform does have the virtue of addressing the imbalance of the political marketplace in an innovative manner.

In general, one must conclude that enforcement and compliance problems in long-term care will continue to exist despite current reform efforts. These problems are inherent in the regulation of every industry and have shown a remarkable resistance to proposed "solutions." Improved enforcement will occur only when a mechanism is developed that increases the benefits of that effort and concentrates them on specific participants in the regulatory process, thereby creating a more balanced political marketplace for long-term care regulation.

NOTES

1. See, for example, K. D. Frank, "Government Support for Nursing Care," *New England Journal of Medicine* 287 (September 14, 1972): 538-545; Joseph Manes, *Federal Programs Providing Long-Term Care to the Aged and Disabled,* Congressional Research Service, Library of Congress (1975).
2. "Nursing-Home Standards Grow Feeble, Toothless," *Medical World News* 10 (September 26, 1969): 24-26.
3. Ibid.
4. R. M. Moroney and N. R. Kurtz, "The Evolution of Long-Term Care Institutions," in *Long-Term Care,* ed. S. Sherwood (New York: Spectrum Publications, 1975): 81-121.
5. E. Bowman, "Support Mounts for Nursing Home Reform," *The Congressional Quarterly,* 94th Congress (1975): 651.
6. See, for example, R. A. Posner, "Theories of Economic Regulation," *Bell Journal of Economics and Management Science* 5 (Autumn 1974): 335-357; G. J. Stigler, "The Theory of Economic Regulation," *Bell Journal of Economics and Management Science* 2 (Spring 1971): 3-21.
7. Posner, "Theories of Economic Regulation."
8. U.S. Congress, Senate, Special Committee on Aging, Subcommittee on Long-Term Care, *Nursing Home Care in the United States: Failure in Public Policy: Nurses in Nursing Homes: The Heavy Burden* [*The Reliance on Untrained and Unlicensed Personnel*] (Washington, DC: Government Printing Office, 1975).
9. U.S. Congress, Senate, Special Committee on Aging, Subcommittee on Long-Term Care, *Nursing Home Care in the United States: Failure in Public Policy* (Washington, DC: Government Printing Office, 1974): 11.
10. R. M. Kemler, "Access to Nursing Homes: A Crisis for Elderly Medicaid Recipients," *Health Law Project Library Bulletin* 318 (University of Pennsylvania, February 1976): 1-7.

11. Roger Noll, "The Consequences of Public Utility Regulation of Hospitals," in *Controls on Health Care* (Washington, DC: Institute of Medicine, National Academy of Sciences, 1975), pp. 25-48.

12. Anthony Downs, *An Economic Theory of Democracy* (New York: Harper & Row, 1957).

13. T. R. Marmor, D. A. Wittman, and T. C. Heagy, "The Politics of Medical Care Inflation," *Journal of Health Politics, Policy and Law* 1 (Spring 1976): 69-84.

14. Kemler, "Access to Nursing Homes: A Crisis for Elderly Medicaid Recipients."

15. Ibid.

16. Jon B. Christianson, "Balancing Policy Objectives in Long-Term Care," *Health Services Research* (Summer 1978): 157-170.

17. M. A. Mendleson and D. Hapgood, "Political Consequences of Aging—The Political Economy of Nursing Homes," *Annals of the American Academy of Political and Social Science* 415 (September 1974): 95-105.

18. D. Shulman and R. Galanter, "Reorganizing the Nursing Home Industry," *Milbank Memorial Fund Quarterly* 54 (Fall 1976): 129-143.

19. G. J. Stigler, "The Optimum Enforcement of Laws," *Journal of Political Economy* 78 (May/June 1970): 526-536.

20. Nationally, approximately 30 percent of long-term care facilities are nonprofit, while 58 percent of the facilities in the sample fit this classification.

21. Ball has argued that one of the important, but often neglected, functions of any regulatory enforcement process should be the dissemination of information about noncompliance to consumers so that they might make more informed purchase decisions. See Robert M. Ball, "Background of Regulation in Health Care," *Controls on Health Care* (Washington, DC: Institute of Medicine, National Academy of Sciences, 1975): 3-32.

22. The assumption is that the compliance with regulatory standards (as measured by the inspection process) *causes* increased expenses.

23. Theil has demonstrated that the use of this technique is redundant when the same matrix of values for the independent variables is employed in estimating each equation in the system. Therefore a two-stage estimator was not used as an alternative to least squares for the income and expense equations of Table 7.4. See H. Theil, *Principles of Econometrics* (New York: John Wiley, 1971), p. 302.

24. W. J. Bicknell and D. C. Walsh, "Perspectives on Long-Term Care: Regulation, Resource Allocation, and Social Policy," paper presented at the 103rd Meeting of the American Public Health Association (November 19, 1975).

25. H.S. Ruchlin, S. Levey, and C. Muller, "The Long-Term Care Marketplace: An Analysis of Deficiencies and Potential Reform by Means of Incentive Reimbursement," *Medical Care* 13 (December 1975): 979-1000.

26. Shulman and Galanter, "Reorganizing the Nursing Home Industry," p. 129.

27. Ibid., p. 141.

28. Jon B. Christianson, "Contracts and Nursing Homes: Comments on a Reform Proposal," Staff Paper 77-10, Department of Agricultural Economics and Economics, Montana State University, 1977.

Chapter 8

Representing Consumer Interests
Imbalanced Markets, Health Planning, and the HSAs

The passage of the National Health Planning and Resources Development Act of 1974, PL 93-641, set in motion the establishment of 205 health systems agencies (HSAs) across the country. The aims of the legislation were ambitious—to produce planning "with teeth," to cut the costs of medical care, to rationalize access, and to do so with more attention to consumer interests than was the case under earlier health planning. Many commentators expected these efforts to produce little change. Yet in some state and local areas the tasks of health planning have been taken up with fervor. Our interest is the connection between consumer representation and these health planning institutions. Our focus is on the conceptual, legal, and administrative questions raised by efforts to create HSA boards dominated by actors "broadly representative" of the constitutents of each local HSA. Our aim is to untangle some of the theoretical and political difficulties that have bedeviled PL 93-641's efforts to improve consumer representation.

We first set a broad theoretical background, and show why concentrated interests (such as medical care providers) dominate the politics of most industries. Representing consumers is

Authors' Note: *From Theodore R. Marmor and James A. Morone, "Representing Consumer Interests: Imbalanced Markets, Health Planning, and the HSAs,"* Milbank Memorial Fund Quarterly/Health and Society, *Vol. No. 1 (Winter 1980), pp. 125-162. Copyright © 1980 by Milbank Memorial Fund and Massachusetts Institute of Technology. Reprinted by permission.*

The authors want to thank Brian Barry particularly for his careful reading and constructive criticisms. Various other colleagues at the Institution for Social and

cast as an important attempt to break this recurring pattern in decision-making about public choices.

In the core of the chapter, we analyze the concept of representation and such associated notions as accountability and participation. Understanding these concepts is important in explaining why the law's clumsy efforts at representing consumers have fostered legal challenges and will almost certainly continue to fail. We describe a number of these failures and prescribe in brief outline a remedy that seems conceptually more defensible and legally more practical.

It would be naive, nonetheless, to expect the Health Planning Act to achieve a major reorientation in American medicine, even if consumer representation were successfully instituted. We suggest reasons why this should be so, emphasizing the wildly inflated expectations characterizing PL 93-641 and its rhetorical promises about planning's high technology and regulatory "teeth."

Our effort throughout is to describe, illuminate, and appraise one widely discussed policy strategy for controlling contemporary medical care: local planning agencies dominated by consumer representatives. While we discuss consumer representation, its potential and limits, current pitfalls and proposed adjustments, we are keenly aware that the health planning law is in flux, that we are appraising, so to speak, a moving target. But, if our analysis is correct, the movements toward controlling medicine through planning and consumer control are crippled by flaws in both the statute and the regulations. Explaining why that is so constitutes this chapter's aim.

Policy Studies, Yale University, and the Center for Health Administration Studies, University of Chicago, have been challenging, and helpful. And our thinking was advanced, particularly at the outset, by the writings and comments of Rudolf Klein and Charles Anderson. Julie Greenberg deserves great credit for improving the successive drafts of this article.

Earlier versions of the chapter were presented at seminars at Yale, Harvard, and the University of Chicago; the penultimate draft was read at the American Political Science Association's Convention, 1979. The topics here discussed are more fully dealt with in part of Morone's dissertation on "Consumer Representation, Public Planning and Democratic Theory."

Representation and Imbalanced Political Markets

The puzzles of representation are exacerbated in circumstances that stimulate representation without explicitly structuring it—when there are no elections, no clearly defined channels of influence, or only murky conceptions of constituency. The politics of regulatory agencies or regional authorities provide examples. Though representatives of groups commonly press their interests within such contexts, there are no systematic canvasses of the relevant interests, such as geographically based elections provide. It is unclear who legitimately merits representation, how representation should be organized, or how it ought to operate.

Interest-group theorists address the problems of representation in precisely such political settings. In their view, interests that are harmed coalesce into groups and seek redress through the political system. Despite the absence of electoral mechanisms of representation, their conception of representation is systematic; every interest that is strongly felt can be represented by a group. At their most sanguine, group theorists suggest that "all legitimate groups can make themselves heard at some crucial stage in the decision-making process."[1] Politics itself is characterized by legions of groups, bargaining on every level of government about policies that affect them. Government is viewed as the bargaining broker, policy choices as the consequences of mutual adjustments among the bargaining groups.[2]

The group model is now partially in eclipse among academic political scientists.[3] One criticism is significant here: Groups that organize themselves for political action form a highly biased sample of affected interests. This argument recalls Schattschneider's[4] classic epigram: "The flaw in the pluralist heaven is that the heavenly chorus sings with a strong upper-class accent. Probably about 90 percent of the people cannot get into the pressure system." Furthermore, that bias is predictable and recurs on almost every level of the political process. We refer to it as a tendency toward imbalanced political markets.

Political markets are imbalanced in part because organizing for political action is difficult and costly. Even if considerable benefits are at stake, potential beneficiaries may choose not to pursue them. If collective goods are involved (that is, if they are shared among members of a group, regardless of the costs any one member paid to attain them, like clean air or a tariff), potential beneficiaries often let other members of the collectivity pay the costs, and simply enjoy the benefits—the classic "free-rider" problem.

Free riders aside, the probability of political action can be expected to vary with the incentives. If either the benefits or the costs of political action are concentrated, political action is more likely. A tax or a tariff on tea, for example, clearly and significantly affects the tea industry. To tea consumers, the tax is of marginal importance, a few dollars a year perhaps. Clearly, those in the industry, with their livelihood at issue, are more likely to organize for political action. And even such concentrated interests are not likely to act if the expected benefits do not significantly outweigh the costs. As Wilson[5] has phrased it, "The clearer the material incentives of the organization's member, the more prompt, focused and vigorous the action."[6] From Tocqueville to David Truman, observers of American politics have argued that threats to occupational status are the most common stimulants to political action. If the group model overstated the facility and extent of group organization, some of its proponents isolated the most significant element: narrow, concentrated producer interests are more likely to pay the costs of political action than broad, diffuse consumer interests.

Not only do concentrated interests have a larger incentive to engage in political action, but they also act with two significant advantages. First, they typically have ongoing organizations, with staff and other resources already in place. This dramatically lowers the marginal cost of political action. Second, most economic organizations have an expertise that rivals that of other political interests, even government agencies and regulators. Their superior grasp (and sometimes even monopoly) of relevant information easily translates into political influence.

The more technical an area, the more powerful the advantage, but it is almost always present to some extent.

In sum, two phenomena work to imbalance political markets: unequal interests and disproportionate resources. The two are interrelated: Groups with more at stake will invest more to secure an outcome. However, the distinction warrants emphasis, for it has important policy implications. Attempts to stimulate countervailing powers, by making resources available to subordinate groups, are doomed to fail if they do not account for differing incentives to employ them. For example, even a resource such as equal access to policymakers—now the object of considerable political effort—is meaningless if the incentives to utilize it over time are grossly unequal. The reverse case—equal interests, unequal resources—is too obvious to require comment. But that clarity should not obscure the fact that imbalanced markets pose an even greater dilemma than the obvious inequality of group resources.

Naturally, diffuse interests are not always somnolent. There are purposive as well as material incentives to political action. A revolt against a sales tax might necessitate cuts in programs that benefit specific groups—scattered taxpayers defeating concentrated beneficiaries; tea drinkers may be swept into political action (even to the point of dumping the tea into Boston harbor). Both are examples of diffuse interests uniting for political action. Such coalitions tend to be loosely organized and are characterized by a grass-roots style of politics. Since sustained, long-term political action requires careful organization, they tend to be temporary. With the end of a legislative deliberation, the group disbands or sets out in search of new issues. Concentrated interests, however, carry on, motivated by the same incentives that first prompted political action.

The conception of imbalanced political markets is relevant to any level of government, but it is particularly appropriate in considering administrative agencies and bureaus. The problem is less nettlesome for legislatures. On a practical level, lobbying legislators appears only marginally effective; analysts have generally found that politicians are more likely to follow their own opinions or the apparent desires of their constituencies.[7] More important, there is at least a formal representation of every citizen. Of course, this does not minimize the complexities of electoral representation. But elective systems do afford a systematic canvass of community sentiment, however vague a guide it may be to concrete policy.

The advantages of organized groups—whatever their extent in legislative politics—increase after a policy's inception. Such groups can be expected to pursue the policy through its implementation and administration. Administrative politics are far less visible; they are not bounded by clear, discrete decisions and are cluttered with technical details rather than with the symbols that are more likely to arouse diffuse constituencies. The policy focus of program administration is dispersed—temporally, conceptually, even geographically. Only concentrated groups are likely to sustain the attention necessary to participate.

Furthermore, when a bureau deals with a group or an industry over time, symbiotic relationships tend to form. A considerable literature documents the range of these clientele relationships and offers the following account of their life cycle: The industry groups typically have information vital to governing; their cooperation is often necessary to program success; and, as a bureau loses public visibility, the groups with concentrated stakes form a major part of its environment, applying pressure, representing their interests, interacting regularly with the agency.[8]

In extreme cases, groups with intense, concentrated stakes can use a friendly agency to recoup legislative defeats. Important decisions are made in agencies and bureaus that define, qualify, even subvert original legislative intent. Administrative processes may even grow biased to the point that other affected parties are shut out from deliberations that concern them. For example, Congress included a consumer-participation provision in the Hill-Burton Act, but the implementing agency never wrote regulations for it. When consumers overcame the imbalance of interests and sued for participation, they were denied standing. Since the regulations had never been written, consumer representatives had no entry into the policymaking process.[9]

As governmental administration becomes more important, the imperative of balancing political markets becomes more pronounced. The difficulties of doing so are intensified by the disaggregated character of the American political process. In contrast to the British case,[10] congressional oversight of the regulatory and administrative agencies has in the past been uneven and often quite loose. This pattern illustrates imbalanced political markets and its extreme manifestation, agency "capture." The notoriously weak and undisciplined political parties in America contribute to this centrifugal tendency of authority within national government.[11]

The issue we address is how to balance political markets in administrative politics. How do we represent broad, diffuse interests, when all the incentives point to domination by a minority of intensely interested producers? The following discussion analyzes the details of the effort to achieve this balance in local health planning according to the strictures of the 1974 law and subsequent regulation: agencies governed by representative boards ostensibly dominated by consumers. We suggest how clearly understanding and properly institutionalizing the concept of representation can help formulate measures to overcome the tendencies toward imbalance that would normally subvert such efforts.

Consumer Representation and HSAs

The Health Planning Act addressed the issue of interest imbalance by mandating consumer majorities on HSA governing boards: Between 51 and 60 percent of each board must be composed of "consumers of health care . . . broadly representative of the social, economic, linguistic, and racial populations" and of "the geographic areas" of the health service area.[12] The rest of the governing board is to be composed of health care providers. There was no means specified for conforming to this mandate in either the law or the regulations.

Administrators quickly discovered that achieving meaningful consumer representation requires considerably more than simply calling for it. Within two years of the law's enactment, a spate of lawsuits had been filed as various groups contended that they were not being represented; the law's ambiguity lent some plausibility to the claim of almost every group. Equally problematic was the question of who should count as representative of whom. And there were reports of public meetings attended only by providers, of consumers shut out of all meaningful deliberations, and of representatives overwhelmed by technical details.[13] Such difficulties in the efforts to represent consumers were a major factor in the unexpected delays in certification ("full designation") of most agencies; confusion about or repudiation of consumer dominance has actually led to decertification in several instances. Not all the agencies have experienced such troubles, but where HSA success has been achieved, it occurs despite the federal law and its regulations.

Establishing representation requires making fundamental choices. Decisions must be made about the selection of representatives, what those representatives should be like, and the expectations that govern their behavior. Furthermore, the governmental structures within which representatives operate must be considered. Do they encourage or impede effective representation? Is the tendency toward political imbalance redressed? Finally, there is the issue of who is to be represented, a question particularly significant when geographic representation is supplemented or abandoned.

The character and success of consumer representation is contingent on how these questions get answered. Indeed, many of the difficulties that plague the Health Planning Act follow from a failure even to consider most of them.

Conceptual Puzzles and Consumer Representation

Three factors, central to consumer involvement in PL 93-641, have been conceptually muddled, both in the law itself and in the analysis and litigation surrounding it. They are accountability, participation, and representation.

Accountability. Put simply, accountability means "answering to" or, more precisely, "having to answer to." One must answer to agents who control the scarce resources one desires. In the classic electoral example, officials are accountable to voters because they control the scarce resources officials desire. Public officials are accountable to legislatures, which control funds; to pressure groups, who can extend or withdraw support; or even to medical providers, who can choose whether to cooperate with an official's program.

The crucial element in each case is that accountability stems from some resource valued by the accountable actor. Accountability is thus not merely an ideal—such as honesty—that public actors "ought" to strive toward. Rather, the resources one cares about hang in the balance, controllable by the relevant constituency.

We call the means by which actors are held to account "mechanisms of accountability." These mechanisms can vary enormously in character and in the extent of control they impose on an actor. For example, voters can occasionally exert control with a yes or no decision, whereas work supervisors can regularly monitor a subordinate's work, enforcing compliance with specific demands.

There is often, to be sure, a give-and-take process in which actors try to maximize their freedom of action within the constraints of the formal mechanisms and thus minimize accountability. And those indifferent to the scarce resources in question (such as an official who has no desire to be reelected) are not, strictly speaking, accountable. But this illustrates the crucial point: In speaking of accountability one must be able to point to specific scarce resources, particular mechanisms that hold representatives to account.

Many of the HSA requirements that are touted as increasing accountability to the public are, in fact, irrelevant to it: a public record of board proceedings;[14] open meetings, with the notice of meetings published in two newspapers and an address given where a proposed agenda may be obtained;[15] an opportunity to comment, either in writing or in a public meeting, about designation,[16] or health system plans (HSPs),[17] or annual implementation plans (AIPs).[18]

These requirements might be said to facilitate public accounting, not accountability. Public participation and information can inform the exercise of accountability but, without formal mechanisms that force boards to answer to consumers, there is not what we call direct public accountability.

Well-defined mechanisms of accountability are central to the idea of holding leaders to account. Propositions that substitute such notions as "winning over" or "working with" the community for an identifiable mechanism are much weaker, conflating the common-language usage of accounting for action with accountability to a constituency, a distinction pointed out by our colleague, Douglas Yates.

Suggesting that health systems agencies would be ineffective without public support is an equally weak conception of accountability to consumers. Every agency of every government expresses these expectations and fears. What is unique about representative government is that the citizenry—not the government agencies—is given the final say. And that say is not expressed by "inhospitality" or "lack of trust" or "written protests" but by an authoritative decision. What we term mechanisms of accountability are the institutionalization of that authoritative decision.

Accountability can be to more than one constituency. As health planning is now structured, the Department of Health, Education, and Welfare (HEW), state governments, local governments, consumers, providers, and numerous other groups can all attempt to hold an HSA accountable. These competing agents introduce significant tensions. One especially difficult problem is the conflict between accountability to local and to national government. There are indications that precisely this conflict is asserting itself as HEW, for example, drafts guidelines, and local communities protest that they do not apply in their specific situations. (Rudolf Klein has elaborated this argument in the British context, with elegant insight on the question of consumer participation.[19])

The emphasis on community control rests on Jeffersonian traditions, and has been seized upon by opponents of big government and centralized bureaucracies. Local communities, according to this view, understand their own needs best and ought, therefore, to be responsible for the policies by which they are governed.

The opposing position draws from sources as disparate as Marx and Weber, Madison and Hamilton. National needs require national solutions. What is good for individual communities (for example, the best hospitals) may not sum to what is best for the entire nation (lower medical costs). This conception typically expresses egalitarian values—only a national policy can redistribute costs and benefits among states and regions.

Accountability in the Health Planning Act is only partially delineated, and is therefore geographically ambiguous. Since local communities establish their agency's modus operandi, the potential for local accountability is present. However, insofar as the law takes up the issue explicitly, it presses accountability to HEW.

HEW is responsible for reviewing the plans, the structure, and the operation of every designated agency at least once every twelve months (sec. 201515 [c] [1]). Presumably, renewal of designation (an important resource that HSA boards desire) is at stake. This is accountability in every important sense. But it can be traced to the public only through the long theoretical strand leading through the presidency. From this perspective, HSA boards are no more accountable to the public than is any other executive agency—certainly a far cry from the rhetoric that accompanied the enactment of PL 63-641. As the law now stands, accountability to the public (either directly or through states and localities) is not prohibited or rendered impossible. But neither is accountability to the public instituted or even significantly facilitated.

Participation. In classical political thought, self-government meant direct participation by the citizenry in public decisions. In this context, Plato envisioned a republic small enough for an orator to address; Aristotle, one in which each citizen could know every other. Rousseau argued that democracy ended when participation did. For obvious reasons, such formulations are generally considered anachronisms in modern industrial societies. Representation has replaced direct participation as the institutionalization of the idea that "every man has the right to have a say in what happens to him".[20] From a theoretical perspective, it is surprising that a law as concerned with consumer representation as PL 93-641 articulates so few guidelines regarding representation, and so many regarding direct public participation.

The earlier discussion of imbalanced political markets suggests why direct participation provisions tend to favor providers over consumers. First, their interest in health planning is far more concentrated and obvious. Planning decisions can directly affect their livelihood. Hospital administrators, officials of state medical associations, and other employed medical care personnel are far more likely to pay the costs of participating in open HSA meetings. The general public—"the consumers"—are not likely to do so. After all, their stake in the proceedings is much smaller; planning does not usually affect their livelihood in as obvious a way.

Furthermore, the difficulties of fostering direct consumer participation are aggravated by the nature of health issues. Health concerns, though important, are intermittent for most people. They are not as clearly or regularly salient as the condition of housing or children's schools—situations that citizens confront daily. Consequently, it is far more difficult to establish public participation in HSAs than in renters' associations or school districts.[21]

We are not suggesting that provisions for participation are objectionable or should be stricken from PL 93-641. Rather, without being carefully tied to some mechanism of accountability or broader view of representation, the provisions are, at best, marginally useful to consumers. They are most likely to be utilized by aroused provider institutions.

Representation. Representation is necessitated by the impossibility of direct, participatory democracy in modern society. The entire population cannot be present to make decisions. Hence, institutions must be designed to "represent"—literally, "to make present again" or to "make present in some sense something which is nevertheless not present literally or in fact."[22]

Three aspects of representation are usually considered in the appraisal of representative institutions: formal, descriptive, and substantive features, a formulation originated by Griffiths[23] and refined and popularized by Pitkin.[24]

By *formal representation* we mean the institutionalization of representation—the specific mechanisms by which representatives are selected and controlled. The mechanisms need have nothing to do with what representatives should be like (descriptive) or the way in which they should act (substantive). Yet they are crucial in defining the process of representation. They are the structure through which representation is established and carried on; they define constituencies and link representatives to them. Institutionalizing accountability rests in large measure on formal requirements.

One commonsense definition of representation is purely formal. Birch,[25] for example, suggests that "the essential character of political representatives is the manner of their selection, not their behavior or characteristics or symbolic value." To him, elections equal representation. Few theorists would agree to so starkly formal a view. More commonly, elections must not merely be held but must offer significant "choice"—they must be "free."[26] Although empirical referants are often noted (elections in the UK, not in the USSR), theorists have had difficulty in specifying precisely what constitutes "free" elections.

The most important issue of formal representation relevant to PL 93-641 is whether representatives should be selected in general elections, by organized groups, by officials, or by self-selection. Though in many cases accountability to the community is increased by general elections, we do not believe that is the case for HSAs.

The Health Planning Act leaves most formal representational questions to be answered on the local level. This is not necessarily unfortunate, as long as the applications for designation are carefully reviewed regarding the issues of formal representation. These issues can be stated in broad terms by asking what constituency a representative is tied to, and by what institutional arrangements.

Descriptive representation refers to the characteristics of representatives. Early formulations of representation held that, since constituencies could not be present themselves to make public choices, they should be "represented" by a "body which [is] an exact portrait, in miniature, of the people at large." The reasoning is straightforward. Since not all the people can be present to make decisions, representative bodies ought to be miniature versions or microcosms of the public, mirroring the populations they represent. The similarity of composition is expected to result in similarity of outcomes; the assembly will "think, feel, reason (and, therefore) act" as the public would have (John Quincy Adams).[27]

A number of difficulties confront this formulation. First, "the public" is a broad entity. What aspect of it ought to be reflected in an assembly? The map metaphor is telling in this regard: Do we want the kind of map that shows rainfall, or altitudes? Topography? Trade regions? Dialects?

John Stuart Mill argued that opinions should be represented; Bentham and James Mill emphasized subjective interests; Sterne, more ambiguously, "opinions, aspirations and wishes"; Burke, broad fixed interests. Swabey suggested that citizens were equivalent units, that if all had roughly equal political opportunities, representatives would be a proper random selection and, consequently, would be descriptively representative. Whichever the case, a failure to specify precisely what characteristics are mirrored reduces microcosm or mirror theories to incoherence.

Even when the relevant criterion for selecting representatives is properly specified, mirroring an entire nation is chimerical. Mill's "every shade of opinion," for example, cannot possibly be reconstructed in the assembly hall on one issue, much less on all. One cannot mirror a million consumers, no matter which sixteen or eighteen consumers are representing them on the HSA governing board. Competing opinions or interests can, of course, be represented. But the chief aim of microcosmic representation is mirroring the full spectrum of constituencies. Pitkin notes that the language in which these theories is presented indicates the difficulty of actually implementing them. The theorists constantly resort to metaphor—the assembly as map, mirror, portrait. They are all unrealistic in more practical terms.

Mirroring the populace may be as undesirable as it is infeasible. Many opinions are idiotic. The merriment that followed Senator Hruska's proposal that the mediocre deserved representation on the U.S. Supreme Court suggests a common understanding of the foolishness of baldly descriptive views.[28]

Furthermore, if representatives are asked merely to reflect the populace, they have no standards regarding their behavior as representatives. Descriptive representation tells us only what representatives are, not what they do. Opinion polls would be more appropriate mechanisms for identifying public views.

Though microcosm theories are neither realistic nor achievable, descriptive (if not precisely mirror) views are relevant to the operation of modern legislatures. Legislators are commonly criticized for not mirroring their constitutents' views or interests. In fact, Adams's formulation might be recast as one guideline to selecting representatives—members of the public vote, essentially, for candidates who appear to "think, feel, reason, and act" as they do. Thus, descriptive qualities inform the operation of formal mechanisms. But surely such very generally conceived descriptive representing is entirely different from the utopian endeavor of forming a microcosm of the populace in the assembly hall.

One contemporary manifestation of microcosm views is what Greenstone and Peterson[29] refer to as "socially descriptive representation." Rather than mirroring opinions or interests, this conception proposes mirroring the social and demographic characteristics of a community's population. A precarious link is added to Adams's already rickety syllogism: If people (a) share demographic characteristics, (b) they will "think, feel, and reason" like one another and, consequently,

(c) act like one another. This is both bad logic and pernicious to the substantive representation of consumer interests.

The problems with mirror views, enumerated above, are all relevant to this version. Demographically mirroring a populace in an assembly is even more unlikely than mirroring their opinions. Obviously, not all social characteristics can (or ought to) be represented; the problem of discriminating among them is particularly vexing. Common sense rebels at representing lefthanders or redheads. What of Lithuanians? Italians? Jews? The uneducated? Mirror views provide no guidelines for drawing such distinctions. Their central conception—the microcosm—is flawed, impossible. It is necessary to look beyond the logic of descriptive representation to choose the social groups that ought to be represented.

Even when the categories to be mirrored are specified, problems remain. Not all individual members of a social group will, in fact, "think, feel, and reason" alike; and they will not act with equal efficacy. Yet, in itself, mirror representation does not distinguish among members of a population group—one low-income representative, for example, is interchangeable with any other. As long as the requisite number of a population group is seated, the society is represented—mirrored—in the appropriate aspect. Such actors are not truly representatives but are mere instances of population groups.

Socially descriptive representation is pernicious because it removes the necessity of recourse to the constituency. The need for formal selection mechanisms and accountability is obviated. Skin color or income, for example, marks a representative as acceptable or not acceptable, regardless of what the constituency thinks. The result is that any member of the group is as qualified a representative as any other. This is a situation that almost begs for "tokenism." If the only requirement is that a fixed percentage of the board must be drawn from a certain group, there is nothing to recommend blacks, elected by fellow blacks or selected by NAACP, or women, elected by women or selected by NOW, over blacks and women "drafted" onto a board because they will "not rock the boat." Precisely this logic operated in New York litigation (*Aladmuy* v. *Pirro,* discussed below), where the judge found that, as long as the "quota" of minorities and poor was filled, there was nothing for him to do. He would not distinguish among them.

It has been suggested that socially descriptive representation might be effective if the representatives were tied to the groups they represented by some kind of pressure, some sort of oversight. Such representation then moves beyond mere socially descriptive representation. The selected agent is then a representative, not merely as an instance of a group's features, but because he or she is acceptable to that group. Thus, we return to a formal conception of representation—the constituency selecting a representative who "thinks, feels, reasons, and acts" as it does.

PL 93-641, as it currently stands and has been interpreted in the New York and Texas district-court cases, does not provide for this. It requires only that the composition of the board be a statistical microcosm of the constituency's racial, sexual, and income distribution. The Health Planning Act does attempt to expand the health role of often-overlooked groups. But, to be successful, it must mandate more than proportional representation on the HSA board; it must require that groups select and monitor their representatives.

Still, for all its difficulties, there is a kernel of truth (as Birch points out) within the theory of socially descriptive representation. Often social categories are related to interests; and, as we will argue in the following section, interests are what ought to be represented. Thus, religious affiliation bespeaks definite interests in Northern Ireland, race affects interests in America, poverty defines specific interests everywhere. And although the actual representation of interests may be subtle and complicated to evaluate, the social categories that are attached to them are almost correspondingly easy.

The choices regarding formal and descriptive representation must be made with the objective of furthering genuinely representative behavior, or *substantive representation*. This is an analytic category by which representatives can be guided and evaluated.

The central question about representative behavior is whether it is in the interest of the constituency. This raises the hoary problem of defining "interest."[30] Is it to be understood as objective fact or subjective choice? The answer determines whether representatives should be considered "messengers," simply conveying constituent desires and acting on constituent requests, or "guardians," doing what the representatives consider to be in the constituents' interest, without consulting them. Substantive representation fits neither of these extremes. Though certain choices are surely in a constituency's objective interest, regardless of their opinions, liberal institutions are ultimately structured on consent. Representatives may pursue their own understanding of constituent interest, but at some point the constituency must make a judgment. The directness of the judgment depends on the formal representation mechanisms, but that there is judgment is crucial.

There is always a danger of drift from substantive representation to simply a guardian or messenger role. In PL 93-641, the former can occur, for example, when an organized group selects a representative and exerts too much control over his or her behavior. But drifting toward the guardian role is the greatest danger for consumer representatives.

Health issues are often viewed as technically complex; PL 93-641 encourages that view in its emphasis on expert scientific planning. If consumer representatives are to be successful, they will need to develop expertise regarding health and planning issues, either through interaction with the HSA staff or by other means. However, as consumer representatives become sophisticated, their tendency may be to drift toward a guardian role, defending a consumer interest that is thought to be incomprehensible to the consumer constituency. This development may be aggravated when the perception of crisis gives representatives more latitude, at the expense of representational ideals such as accountability.

A related issue is the identity of the constituency. Should governing board representatives be working for the good of the community as a whole? of the consumers as taxpayers? of all black (female, poor) consumers? Some answers may be implicit in the formal mechanisms. The general model underlying HSA boards implicitly follows the liberal ideal of getting all the narrow, self-interested parties together and making them thrash out policy choices among themselves. Each representative works for his or her narrow interest group; yet, through the compromise and bargaining necessary to get the group anything, answers acceptable to all will emerge. If this is the model, then it is important that all groups be in on the bargaining process.

When, for example, lawyers for one HSA emphasize the importance of getting a board that is not segmented, they are incorrect. Ironically, the model calls for a highly segmented, even contentious, board, for a board on which every health interest is vigorously represented will be more contentious than one that is captured or dominated by a single interest.

It is also important that representatives affect policy outcomes. All representatives have some symbolic function; but insofar as they have no other, they are not substantively representative, for they give the public they represent no say over policy.[31]

By this logic it is clear how some representatives can represent their constituencies better than others: they not only perceive what is good for—in the interest of—their constituencies, but also have the ability to act successfully on that perception. An eloquent speaker, a successful operator, a person who is not easily duped, an individual with important contacts or serving on important committees, therefore provides more substantive representation than one with the same opinions but without the same capacities. There are many relevant examples from the community action programs (CAPs) of precisely this phenomenon—boards that were relatively more successful because of the political skills, experience, and intelligence of some of their members[32]

A representative's effectiveness, then, generally flows from a mixture of position and ability. An able person may affect policy, even from a relatively weak position. An incompetent one may fail to do so, even in a position of authority. The point is that substantive representation necessitates both knowing and successfully pursuing the constituents' interests.

Conceptual Puzzles Reconsidered. Substantive representation is the effective pursuit of the interests of the constituency. Ultimately it is the goal of all democratic representation. However, the final judge of representation must be the represented; either directly or indirectly the represented must control some scarce resource their representative wants (votes, for example). Only then can we properly speak of a governing board as accountable to its constituency.

The Health Planning Act gives these issues little consideration. There is no systematically mandated accountability and little evidence of it as a concern. A representative's orientation is considered only in terms of socially descriptive representation. This approach patronizes the relevant groups. It will ineffectively advance consumer representation unless it is linked to effective mechanisms of accountability by which the members of those groups can evaluate the substantive quality of the representation received.

Effective Consumer Representation

This section suggests ways in which adequate consumer representation can be facilitated and effective mechanisms of accountability created. The task, as pointed out earlier, is balancing the health planning political market, rather than just getting consumers on boards.

The HSA staffs are one resource that could help consumers achieve political parity. Staffs generally have considerable expertise in issues of medical care and health. Occupying full-time positions in health planning, they have a concentrated interest in the industry. Is there any reason to believe that they will typically support consumers when there are conflicts of interest?

The evidence thus far shows wide variation in staffs' views. In New England, some play an outspoken proconsumer role.[33] In many other areas they have allied with providers, often seriously undermining consumer representatives who cannot match the combined expertise of providers and staff.[34] Generally the support of the staff appears to be essential to an active consumer role on HSA boards. The problem is systematically harnessing the staffs' market-balancing potential to consumer interests.

The most direct approach is to restructure the health systems agencies so that part of the professional staff is placed under consumer control—to be selected by and accountable to them. The staff's tasks could be specified in any number of ways, but its critical function would be providing professional (expert, full-time) support to the consumer effort.

Another potential for balancing the health planning market lies in organizations that already exist within the consumer population. Political scientists generally agree that the "basic units . . . of polity or political process are groups formed around interests."[35]

The very existence of these groups attests to a commitment to improve the life circumstances of some part of the population. Furthermore, they have already paid the costs of organizing. We can expect their attention to issues to be high and relatively sustained. They can often overcome lack of expertise by redeploying their staffs.[36]

Organizations can meet a problem with more resources and in a more sustained way than isolated individuals. It is telling that much of the litigation challenging HSA boards comes from organizations formed to further the rights or general circumstances of certain disadvantaged groups within the consumer population. Existing "reform" organizations have potential, then, for balancing the health care political market; we believe that they can play an effective role in selecting and monitoring consumer representatives.

The experience of the community action program (CAP) provides some support for this claim. Selection by groups tended to produce the most independent and competent boards. Moreover, where more than one organization wanted to select representatives for the same population or interest, elections were held among the groups. Organizations representing the poor in parts of New York City, for example, competed fiercely to gain support of the community—a far cry from the apathy that greeted general elections and the alienation and cynicism that accompanied selection of representatives by officials.[37]

We recommend, therefore, that those charged with selecting members of consumer boards select not the members themselves, but groups organized around health care interests. If more than one group seeks to select a representative for the same interest, a special election would be called. It is crucial that the interests themselves (for example, poverty, race) be specified by HEW. Competition among groups representing an interest is acceptable, even desirable; competition among interests to be represented is not. (The logic of choosing what interests merit representation on HSA boards will be discussed below.)

A potential gap always exists between an interest felt and a group's articulation of that interest; however, groups that have overcome the obstacles to organization are the most likely promoters of a particular interest. Representatives from these groups will have clearly defined constituencies, experience in organizational politics, and resources at their disposal. These attributes will help them both in identifying group interests and in pursuing them, regardless of their other characteristics. (Even minorities suing for represention in Texas were willing to accept whites to represent blacks, for example, if the NAACP selected them.)

The experience of the CAPs indicates that representatives selected in this way tend to be the most able, show a universalistic orientation, and are least likely to be co-opted.

A group can be expected to monitor its representatives more carefully than will the general public. Thus, as long as the representatives are chosen for a fixed term, accountability is increased. Representatives should be allowed to serve out their terms (without recall) so as not to bind them too tightly to the selecting organization,[38] they should be permitted reelection so that they are not bound too loosely.

Ideally, then, the imbalanced political market in health planning will be tempered by two mechanisms, one internal to the health systems agency (staff assigned to the consumer representatives), the other external (selection of representatives by groups). We expect the former to facilitate organization and expertise among the consumer representatives, the latter to improve representation and heighten their accountability.

Of course, in some locations and for some interests it will be impossible to find appropriate groups. In these cases, another, less desirable, mode of selection (or formal representation) will be necessary. We evaluate two others: general election, and selection by officials.

General Elections. Various reform groups have called for election of consumer representatives in a model roughly based on that for the selection of school boards. The surface plausibility of the proposal should not be permitted to obscure its difficulties. One problem with direct election of representatives to HSA boards stems from the failure of most Americans to consider themselves part of an ongoing health care community. They typically seek care sporadically, and do not conceive of health care in terms of local systems. Both factors distinguish health planning from education or housing issues, where specific elections may be more effective.

Evidence from the CAP poverty programs supports the view that elections are problematic; fewer than 3 percent of the eligible population voted for local CAP boards in Philadelphia, fewer than 1 percent voted in Los Angeles. Those who did vote were moved to do so by personal, not policy, considerations. Overwhelmingly, they voted for their neighbors and, presumably, personal acquaintances. The consequent policy formulated by these representatives was, predictably, overwhelmingly particularistic. It helped their friends, not the community or the interests they ostensibly represented. Representatives generated little community interest or support. They tended to be ineffective advocates and operators.

Since the public chooses its health planning representatives directly, the representatives can theoretically be held accountable with relative ease. However, in practice, low incentives and marginal visibility will undermine elections.

It is important to note that "antiparticipation" city officials, who could not control the selection of CAP boards, preferred elections as the alternative. They apparently felt that this formal mechanism would not threaten their interests by generating energetic, aggressive representation of the interests of poor people—an outcome they feared from selection by groups.

Selection by Local Officials. This mechanism leaves accountability to the public very tenuous. The constituency is left with no direct control over its representatives, but must hold the selector of the representatives to account. In the worst cases, the selector is not directly accountable to the public either. Boards selected by local officials are accountable to, and presumably controlled by, local government; they will be as accountable as any other local agency. Yet they operate within a program that promises direct consumer participation. When a health planning issue becomes highly visible, we expect this mismatch of rhetoric and reality to cause public frustration and alienation.

Since officials can choose whichever member of a group they desire, many will choose ones that "make no trouble." Thus descriptive representation (what representatives "think, feel, and reason") will probably be low, even when socially descriptive representation is high.

Substantive representation will generally be low. The HSA, over time, will become indistinguishable from other agencies in the local health care bureaucracy.

Who Should Be Represented?

We now turn from the means of securing effective consumer representation to the issue of who should be represented. Which elements of the consumer population merit health representation?

The notion of dividing up the consumer population for the purpose of representation implies that there are subgroups of the consumer population with distinctive health care interests that ought to be represented.

Only one subcategory has been precisely delineated in PL 93-641—those individuals who live in nonmetropolitan areas. Their representation on the board must reflect the proportion of nonmetropolitan residents in the health service area.[39] As for the rest, PL 93-641 says only that consumers should be "broadly representative of the social, economic, linguistic, and racial population" of the area.[40]

Unscrambling the present confusion about representation requires an assessment of what consumer involvement is intended to accomplish. Presumably, the goal is to facilitate the articulation and satisfaction of the health care needs in American communities. If so, what is required is substantive representation, not hollow tokenism. Different health care interests in the area must be identified and selected for special attention through representation. The reason for including such groups as minorities, low-income persons, and women on the board should not be to mirror the community's population on the boards; that, we have argued, is foolish and impossible. Rather, certain groups—minorities, low-income people, and women—should be included insofar as they have different and important health interests that the political system ought to consider. The argument is most compelling when it refers to interests that are often overlooked in local political processes. Moving from mirror representation to the effort to improve representation of specified interests requires changing the language of the law requiring that consumer representatives be "broadly representative of the . . . populations" of the health service area, to language requiring them to be "representative of consumer health interests" of the health servie area.

The obvious question, then, is what specific consumer health interests should be represented? The answer is not easy because interests vary by issue. Regarding questions of access to health care, the current debate has identified various groups with legitimate claims. For example, access problems are different for rural and for urban populations, or for the chronically as opposed to the intermittently ill. At the same time, there are groups that, while part of the population (and therefore potentially included on a board constituted on the microcosm principle), do not genuinely have health care interests peculiar to their own group. For example, it is not clear that those with little formal education have specific health care needs or interests in the same way as the low-income or the aged populations.

As issues change, so do the interests that claim the right to a spokesperson. The infirm could claim a representative for every type of disease, when the issue of new facilities arises; so could every ethnic group with specific genetic diseases that disproportionately or exclusively afflict them (blacks, Jews, Italians, for instance). The possible list is very long. However, to avoid an infinite round of litigation, HEW must make the difficult choices and specify the various consumer subgroups with recognizable health care interests that ought to be represented on the HSA boards. In this way, the present, almost infinitely broad, mandate would be replaced by one that is highly specific.

To illustrate, HEW could specify that groups reflecting the following interests be provided representation on the HSA board in approximate proportion to their number in the health service area: (a) the poor; (b) women; (c) the aged; (d) racial or linguistic groups comprising significant portions of the population; (e) area of residence (the Codman Report [1977] breaks health service areas into hospital service areas—essentially, these are large catchment areas corresponding to the distribution of hospitals within a health service area. We suggest such a division of all health service areas, getting representatives from each subdivision in approximate proportion to its percentage of the total population of the health service area); (f) groups that pay for medical care, such as insurance companies or unions; (g) other identifiable groups that the secretary of HEW recognizes as having a health care interest and forming a significant segment of the population. Examples are migrant workers, black-lung victims, and persons exposed to occupational hazards. These groups should be specified by the secretary either on the recommendation of the state or by appeal of that group.[41]

The specification of interest we propose will not only curtail the stream of litigation that has sprung from the microcosm view, but will also help ensure the representation of important interests. As the law stands, a great deal of discretion regarding who is represented is left to state and local political games. And while it is appropriate to maximize the competition among groups on the board regarding health care issues, it is important to minimize the competition over which interests get on the board in the first place to compete over these issues. The danger is that groups will try to take over the boards, shutting out other legitimate interests. The vagueness of the current law and regulations as to who is to be represented increased the possibility of conflict—and some of the litigation indicates that fear of further conflict is not groundless.

While the preceding discussion resolves a practical problem, it introduces a theoretical one: There is no systematic rationale by which HEW can make those "difficult choices" among affected interests. No matter which interests are selected, not all individuals are equally represented, or even equally enfranchised. How, under such conditions, can HSAs claim legitimacy as authoritative community decision makers?

The answer is clear when there is a macrotheory of objective interests spanning the entire citizenry, such as class analyses include. However, liberal theory offers no comparable vision of fixed systematic interests. Pluralism brilliantly avoided the issue by assuming the link between subjective interest felt and group formed. Bentley is clear and adamant on this issue: "To state the raw materials of political life[—] the groups directly insisting on [a policy] . . . those directly opposing it, and those more directly concerned in it—is much more complete than any statement in terms of self-interest, theories or ideals".[42] Market conceptions provide little help. Although the populace is, theoretically, divisible into consumers and providers, regarding any functional area, those labels press a horde of often competing interests under a single label. As shown earlier, seating "consumer" representatives is a difficult mandate, regardless of the infelicitous mandate that boards be "broadly representative." Finally, the choices we have urged HEW to make are plausible, not Platonic ones.

This does not mean that we are without a rationale for selecting interests. Emerging groups can be legitimated or strengthened as political actors by this type of quasi-corporatist program. The most important of these may be advocacy groups speaking for broad consumer constituencies and organizations such as unions and industrial associations. They are organized and have a clear, relatively concentrated interest in the politics of medical care. Such groups are promising market balancers. Other interests (minority groups, poverty groups) can be included for similar reasons, or because it is reasonable, necessary, or prudent to include them, given the objectives of the program. Anderson's[43] elaboration of this argument helps clarify the problem of the legitimacy of the HSA boards.

For various reasons, HSAs are structured to improve public accountability and representation. However, that structure is not relevant to the legitimacy of these agencies qua governmental units. HSAs must be viewed as a supplement to, rather than a substitute for, geographic representation. As administrative agencies, their legitimacy flows not from representational schemes, but from a legislative mandate—from Congress.

Litigation and Representation

PL 93-641 was enacted in January 1975. By December 1977, it was the subject of eighteen lawsuits, five of which included the issue of consumer representation. These five cases are analyzed below in light of the preceding discussion of representation and accountability.

Aladmuy et al. v Pirro et al., C.A. No. 76-CV-204 (N.D., N.Y., April 7, 1977). The plaintiffs were dissatisfied with the minority representation on the Syracuse-Onandaga County

(N.Y.) Planning Agency. The court ruled against plaintiffs because the representation of minorities was numerically adequate. With respect to the selection of certain minority members over others, the court stated that it would not find an abuse of discretion by the secretary of HEW except where the secretary's action was "so arbitrary as to be clearly wrong."

The case is an illustration of the application of the new of mirror representation. The court found no criterion in either the law or the regulations by which to judge representatives except for descriptive characteristics (in this case, "minority" status). Since both the representatives selected for the HSA board and their challengers satisfied that criterion, there was no way to choose between them. It was not possible to select one minority group member as any better, or more "representative," than any other. Since PL 93-641 and its regulations say nothing about formal representation, challengers have no recourse and courts have no reason to insist on accountability if the criterion of socially descriptive representation is minimally satisfied.

Three companion cases can be considered together:

The Louisiana Association of Community Organizations for Reform Now (ACORN) et al. v New Orleans Area/Bayou Rivers Health Systems Agency et al., C.A. No. 17-361 (E.D. La., filed March 15, 1977). ACORN is an association of low- to moderate-income citizens claiming that the New Orleans HSA is not "socially or economically" representative of the area. ACORN states that of thirty-nine consumer members of the board, only four have incomes under $10,000.

Rakestraw et al. v Califano et al., C.A. No. C77-635A (N.D. Ga., Atlanta Div., filed April 22, 1977). Plaintiffs assert that there is inadequate representation of low-income individuals and families as well as of the handicapped and women.

Califano is cited, not only for conditionally designating a board with inadequate representation of the above-mentioned groups, but for failing to "propose and promulgate regulations dealing with the composition . . . and selection process" of HSA boards. The court is asked to require Califano to devise a method of selecting consumer representatives that renders them accountable to the public.

Texas ACORN et al. v Texas Area V Health Systems Agency et al., C.A. No. S-76-102-CA (E.D. Texas, Sherman Div., March 1, 1977). The plaintiffs argued that only three of the forty-one consumer representatives have incomes below the median for the area ($10,000). They argued that if people with income above the median are to represent lower-income consumers ("under specific circumstances"), then the burden of proof is on the defendant HSA to indicate how some or all of the board members with over $10,000 incomes would represent the poor.

They contend that representatives of the "public at large" do not count as representatives of the poor; this is a consequence of the model underlying their notion of HSAs, one of pluralistic bargaining among interests.

The federal defendants replied that it is not necessary to be poor to represent the poor; but they conceded that the federal regulations were inadequate, with regard both to the selection of the consumer representatives and to the representation of consumers on the board. (Note that these are precisely the charges in *Rakestraw.*)

The district court(a) enjoined the defendant HSA from acting as an HSA or expending HSA funds, and (b) ruled that between sixteen and twenty-five of the forty-one representatives must have incomes below the mean. Thus a strictly mathematical delineation was made, with a little "give" in it to make it "broadly" rather than "precisely" representative.

Defendant HEW has asked for a stay in the case until regulations can be developed; it will then be determined whether the Texas HSA conforms to the regulations.

Once again we find HEW mired in attempts to enforce socially descriptive representation. In bringing suit, the ACORN organizations use the mirror conception of representation to their advantage. But they recognize that it alone will not suffice to produce adequate representation of consumer interests over the long run. This realization—although present in all three cases—is most explicit in *Rakestraw.* There, HEW is sued not only regarding the "composition" but also regarding the "selection" of boards. The suit asks HEW to consider what we describe as the formal aspect of representation. Furthermore, plaintiffs demand not mere specification of a formal mechanism, but a mechanism that guarantees accountability to the public. They are, to some extent, willing to waive socially descriptive requirements in favor of accountability engendered by the selection process. The tradeoff is illustrated in the Texas ACORN brief, with the suggestion that a white selected by the NAACP would be acceptable from the perspective of black interests.

Texas ACORN et al. v Texas Area Health Service Area et al., 559 F2nd 1019 (U.S. Court of Appeals, 5th Cir., Sept. 23, 1977). On appeal, a broader view of the case was taken. The district court's undifferentiated mirror view was rejected and a full evidentiary hearing, in which HEW demonstrated precisely how board members were representative of the low-income or demographic population, was mandated. The view that one must be a member of those groups was explicitly rejected.

This ruling shows a far greater sensitivity to the issues of representation. There is cognizance of questions regarding the representatives' relations to their constituencies and the necessity of various skills relevant to achieving substantive representation. In sum, there is awareness that a mindless adherence to the mirroring ideal can undermine the effective (or, in our terms, substantive) representation of a constituency's interests.

Amos et al. v Central California Health Systems Agency et al. C.A. No. 76-174 ci (E.D. Calif., filed Sept. 10, 1976). Plaintiffs charged that whites were underrepresented on the board because Fresno and Kern counties were underrepresented. HEW has sent the defendant agency a letter, noting that its governing board is not composed in conformity with the requirements of PL 93-641, so this case will probably not be settled in court. The race issue was not directly dealt with by HEW but subsumed under the criticism that the representation of metroplitan and nonmetropolitan areas was not fixed in exact proportion to the population. About race, HEW said

> only: "The ethnic representation on your board can be reasonably readjusted when you correct its composition in terms of nonmetropolitan/metropolitan distribution."

The *Amos* case illustrates two other difficulties. First, the charge that minorities "captured" this HSA board, as the plaintiffs claimed, points out the distinction between (a) giving contending groups a place on the board to dispute policy questions, and (b) letting groups contend for the places on—or control over—the board. The latter defeats the purpose of representative boards: to allow local consumer interests to thrash out local health issues with each other as well as with providers.

A second difficulty follows directly from the first. Precisely who is being represented is not made clear by a law and regulations that merely mandate broad representation of the "social, economic, linguistic, and racial populations" of the health service area. Who is to determine what is "broadly representive"? We have argued that the concept of "broadly representing" (mirroring) a community is a meaningless guide to consumer representation. Instead, the interests or groups that merit representation must be specified precisely. That specification must be made with a fuller understanding of representation than is at present evident in PL 93-641.

Health Policy, Health Plans, and the HSAs

HSAs face insurmountable problems completely apart from that of representing consumers. The Health Planning Act has generated expectations for reshaping American medicine that no HSA can meet. The health systems agencies are simply not equipped to control inflation, solve problems of inadequate access, or rationalize the health services of a community. In discussing why, we shall point particularly to the factors that were expected to distinguish this planning effort from previous ones—"teeth" and sophisticated technology.

Authority and Health Planning

Serious planning involves choosing goals for the future and the ways of arriving at them. One must distinguish between this sense of planning—manipulating a system toward particular goals in a specified fashion—and the writing of (often unreadable) documents termed "plans." The former requires the capacity for authoritative decisions about the allocation of resources.

How nations in fact plan for health—that is, make allocative decisions regarding future goals—is not exhaustively illuminated (indeed, sometimes not seriously touched on) by studies of how official planning bodies operate. Put another way, we have two subjects: the process of operational health planning, and the process of health planning organizations.[44] The key element is the connection between choosing goals and the capacity to pursue or "implement" them. When the connection is loose—when plans are isolated from the process of resource allocation and, more generally, from authority—planning can become a smokescreen, a symbol, or simply frustrated wheel-spinning.

At the same time, de facto plans will be either the choices of those who in fact allocate resources (the connection between authoritative choices based on financing arrangements and system control holds true under most conditions—including laissez-faire), or a result of the incentives operating within ongoing arrangements. The latter may be termed "change without choice,"[45] but it ought not be confused with the "change without influence" that is implicit in homeostatic—antiplanning—market conceptions. Such arrangements tend to be characterized, not by the theory's self-regulating market, but by the domination of identifiable actors—hospitals, nursing homes, physicians—with an unrelentingly clear incentive: more. Thus, the well-known incentives of an American hospital are more high technology, more modernization, a fuller range of services and, therefore, more prestige, more first-class physicians, and so on. The consequences of this system are impressive technologies, rising costs, and a frustrating lack of corresponding change in health status indicators.[46] An HSA that overcomes some of the problems described above and plans for "less," will need more than its "plan" to deflect that hospital from the incentives that ideology, financing, and provider expectations have generated.

The Amerian suspicion of centralized authority is well documented.[47] Even the sweeping expansion of government legitimacy in the 1930s included only fleeting relaxation of this resistance. Intellectually, the hostility has been expressed in two major ways: in arguments that authoritative planning or control is tyrannous,[48] and that it is not realistic.[49] The Health Planning Act and its HSAs fit obviously into this tradition. Their mission is overstated, their role ambiguous, their authority and political capacity highly circumscribed. They are certainly no match for the grandiosity of their plans. Most of what occurs in local health markets is beyond their jurisdiction: the terms of reimbursement, the closing of facilities, the positive choices of places to expand. The powers they are given are widely qualified: They review certificates of need, but can only make recommendations; they are supposed to conduct "appropriateness review," but the sanctions of inappropriateness are unclear (indeed, the regulations guiding this task remain unpublished).

In sum, HSAs do not have the authority—"teeth" is the current metaphor—necessary for the tasks, such as taming medical inflation, that have been assigned to them.

The difficulties of limited authority are compounded by the uncertain relation between HSAs and the rest of government. Indeed, the brief history of the law reads like a catalogue of contemporary confusions in American federalism: local governments are spurned for the—partially new, partially redundant—HSA structures; states and counties fight for influence within the framework of the law.[50] Federal guidelines are promulgated with little clarity about how seriously they will (or indeed ought to) be taken in the communities. To the confusion of the now traditional "marble cake" metaphor[51] we can add the impermeability of "picket-fence federalism."[52]

Unclearly stated regulations, interagency jealousies, lack of hierarchical support, and a growing, bureaucratic, self-generating political sector[53] lead to confusion, and ineffective governance and planning. Within the confusion, both governmental accountability and authority are dissipated.

We are not sanguine about the HSA successes that have been reported. Logic rebels at the peculiar idea that a planning agency without sufficient authority can scheme, scold, and cajole a dynamic system into compliance with plans that run contrary to all that system's incentives. On their own terms, HSAs will achieve varying levels of success. But they will not achieve the foolish expectations that have been thrust upon them. They simply do not have the authority or the resources.

The Technological Fix

The present health planning effort promised more "teeth" than its failed predecessor (comprehensive health planning), but added few. Another well-publicized innovation was scientific planning. The Health Planning Act was presented as the marriage of community participation and scientific planning. The success of the law was seen to hinge to a large extent on the latter.[54]

The reliance on the technology of planning is the most recent manifestation of a recurring alchemy in American politics: the effort to derive objective solutions from political choices. This impulse was very much a part of the Progressives' search for the "public interest"; relatedly, the "best way" was a kind of grail for scientific managers preoccupied with achieving measurable efficiency.[55]

There are of course legitimate—perhaps pressing—data needs in health delivery. Indeed, data are notoriously poor, and tend to be monopolized by provider institutions, which are predictably reluctant to share them with regulators. And, clear data sometimes have clear policy implications. For example, one Philadelphia study showed that people admitted on Fridays have longer hospital stays than those admitted on Mondays and Tuesdays with the same ailment. Furthermore, a quarter of the hospital days in the same sample were taken up by patients suffering from alcoholic and nervous disorders, both more effectively (and economically) treated on an outpatient basis.[56]

The policy implications of such findings are relatively clear, but difficult to implement. Furthermore, there generally remains the policy leap between facts and political choices—where to build a hospital, how to allocate limited resources, or, more dramatically, "who shall live." Even problems that seem objectively solvable (where to close down hospital beds) are intensely political. Ignoring the realities of political interests and value choices without some fundamental—and unlikely, undesirable—system changes is a naivete that will result in irrelevant plans and frustrated planners.

The difference between data analysis and political choices is reflected in the odd disjunction of commentary on health planning: From Washington and academia flows an apparently steady stream of methodologies, simulations, and data-processing advice. At the same time, reports from the HSAs deal with the different world of power struggles, influence peddling, and political choices. The language of science seems strikingly distant from the realities of local health planners.

There are some fundamental political and philosophical conflicts that the language of technology obscures. Two such conflicts are apparent in the Health Planning Act.

Federalism. The conflict between national demands and local desires was referred to earlier. When a national program invites local participation, the community will generally want to make alterations. Local residents see a different set of needs, for their perspective is different, and community politics—to recall a classic variant—involves a different cast of political actors. The conflict is resolved neatly when de facto responsibility for each part of the program is fixed at one level of government, however much the symbols or rhetoric of the program may distract attention from the outcome.

The structure of the Health Planning Act exacerbates this tension rather than resolving it. The law stimulated wide-ranging community participation, local discretion in agency design, and goals and purposes so vague that they appeared to promise significant local autonomy. However, set expectations, fixed goals, and stringent guidelines followed. With it came a furor that reflected the conflict between local participation and national goals.

Scientific planning cannot relieve this tension. Selecting problems requires choosing between values, as does the series of increasingly narrow decisions that follow. And participants on various levels of government must hammer out agreement about what those choices are. The vision of objective solutions, replicable from place to place (in the manner of scientific experimentation) is, in this context, a vacuous one.

Efficiency. A second formidable conflict lies between representing community interests and program efficiency. The constant juxtaposition of representation and scientific planning reiterates the hope that representative boards can somehow be made efficient with an infusion of "science." In reality, the phrase is an oxymoron—the juxtaposition of opposites.

The point is illustrated nicely by the Common Cause official[57] who was told that his organization was not sufficiently democratic and participatory. He responded that if it were any more so its efficiency at achieving policy objectives would be hampered. He was correct for a number of reasons.

First, inducing wider representation introduces conflict. This may be desirable, indicating the articulation of various interests and perspectives, but it is not administratively efficient. And much of the conflict is irrelevant to the agency's tasks, often reflecting long-standing community animosities, personal agendas, and the like.

Second, the essence of administrative superiority is the skillful gathering, use, and even monopolization of information. Th resulting expertise and technical skills are complicated—often undermined—by the introduction of nonprofessional participants, particularly when they are accountable to outside constituencies rather than to agency superiors. The logic of representation emphasizes a principle directly contrary to the logic of efficient organizational management on this point.

Third, administration will be more time-consuming. Representatives reexamine first questions and basic values; they may need to consult with constituencies, delaying the decision-making process. Such problems particularly complicate long-term planning where objectives must remain fixed over time. The starts and stops of a volunteer-governed agency can make the planning process considerably rougher than one run by professional staff.

The result is that representative institutions are inherently less efficient than bureaucratic ones, even when they are properly institutionalized. In the case of HSAs, the inefficiency is more apparent because amateurs are asked to plan and regulate a technical system that has been highly resistant to almost every sort of government intervention. The litany about marrying representation and science is useless in this regard. It even undermines the HSA effort. For each argument against the efficiency of representation is a hurdle that must be overcome if representation is to survive. And insofar as the myth of science distracts from serious consideration of a proper volunteer role, it contributes to the antirepresentational impulse grounded in the exigencies of efficient administration and planning.

Though expanded interest-representation makes administration less efficient, it is worth pursuing. There are numerous reasons for this choice, though all finally point to the permeability of policymaking institutions by the public.

First, Weber's efficient bureaucracy may not be desirable for policy bodies. The reevaluation of fundamental values, the limitations on technical vocabularies, the brakes on routinization and standard operating procedures, all make such agencies more accessible to public groups.

Furthermore, when limits to bureaucratization are removed, imbalance is facilitated. Bureaucratic agencies tend to tug issues out of politics and resolve them administratively. The bargaining process remains, but entry qualifications grow so high that only concentrated interests are likely to meet them.

Administrators, with their expertise and their specialized vocabulary, grow inscrutable to any but provider (expert) groups. Public accountability is difficult, legislative scrutiny unlikely.

Finally, an open process makes it less likely that groups will be completely shut out—like the consumers suing by participation in Hill-Burton. A market open to all health system actors is more difficult to manage because conflict is introduced; the planning process grows more complicated and time-consuming. However, in a time of dwindling resources, forging a consensus among all health system actors is important to planning success.

In an increasingly bureaucratic age, representation is a more fragile value than efficiency. If the Health Planning Act accomplishes nothing more than introducing and legitimating potential market balancers on an ongoing basis, it will have achieved considerable success.

Conclusion

The vision of representation in the National Health Planning and Resources Development Act is impossibly flawed, but not irretrievably so. We have suggested one plan for achieving reasonably effective consumer representation and balancing provider dominance. But representing consumers, overcoming imbalance, even discerning the public interest in HSAs will not alter the American health system in any profound fashion. The HSA mandate—limiting costs, expanding access, and improving the quality of health—reaches far beyond the agency's capabilities. Measured by these standards, the act's program is trivial, more symbols and rhetoric than significant improvement.

Rather, the law's significance lies in its stimulation of a broad range of consumer interests. Viewed as an effort to organize communities into caring for their own health systems, it is the largest program of its kind. And one that could influence health politics long after its particular institutional manifestations—HSA planning boards—have been forgotten.

NOTES

1. R. Dahl, *A Preface to Democratic Theory* (Chicago: University of Chicago Press, 1964), p. 137.

2. A. Bentley, *The Process of Government* (Cambridge, MA: Harvard University Press, 1967); D. Truman, *The Governmental Process* (New York: Knopf, 1951); R. Dahl, *Who Governs?* (New Haven: Yale University Press, 1961); J. D. Greenstone, "Group Theories," In F. Greenstein and N. Polsby, eds., *The Handbook of Political Science II* (Reading, MA: Addison-Wesley, 1975).

3. A. McFarland, "Recent Social Movements and Theories of Power in America," paper delivered at the American Political Science Convention, Washington, D.C., August 1979; R. Salisbury, "On Centrifugal Tendencies in Interest Systems: The Case of the U.S.," paper delivered at the International Sociological Association, Uppsala, August 17, 1978.

4. E. E. Schattschneider, *The Semisovereign People* (Hinsdale, IL: Dryden, 1960), p. 34.

5. J. Q. Wilson, *Political Organizations* (New York: Basic Books, 1973), p. 318.

6. See also T. R. Marmor, D. Wittman, and T. C. Heagy, "Politics of Medical Inflation," *Journal of Health Politics, Policy and Law* 1(Spring 1976): 69-83.

7. E. E. Schattschneider, *Politics, Pressures and Tariff* (Englewood Cliffs, NJ: Prentice-Hall, 1935); R. A. Baur, I. Pool, and L. A. Dexter, *American Business and Public Policy* (New York: Atherton, 1963); T. R. Marmor, *The Politics of Medicare* (Chicago: Aldine, 1973); H. Eulau and K. Prewitt, *Labyrinths of Democracy* (Indianapolis: Bobbs-Merrill, 1973).

8. M. Bernstein, *Regulating Business by Independent Commission* (Princeton, NJ: Princeton University Press, 1955); R. Noll, *Reforming Regulation* (Washington, DC: Brookings, 1971).

9. R. Rosenblatt, "Health Care Reform and Administrative Law: A Structural Approach," *Yale Law Journal* (1978, part 2): 264-286.

10. G. McConnell, *Private Power and American Democracy* (New York: Knopf, 1966); T. Lowi, *The End of Liberalism* (New York: Norton, 1969).

11. W. D. Burnham, "American Politics in the 1970s: Beyond Party?" in J. Fishel, ed., *Parties and Elections in an Anti-Party Age* (Bloomington: Indiana University Press, 1978).

12. PL 93-641, § 1512(b)(3)(C)(i).

13. W. Clark, "Placebo or Cure? State and Local Health Planning Agencies in the South," Southern Governmental Monitoring Project, Southern Regional Council, Atlanta, 1977.

14. 41 Federal Register 12812 (March 26, 1976), 122.114.

15. 41 Federal Register 12812 (March 26, 1976), 122.104(b)(1)(viii) and 122.109(4)(3).

16. 41 Federal Register 12812 (March 26, 1976), 122.104(a)(8) and 122.104(b)(7).

17. 41 Federal Register 12812 (March 26, 1976), 122.107(c)(2).

18. 41 Federal Register 12812 (March 26, 1976), 122.107(c)(3).
19. R. Klein, "Control, Participation, and the British National Health Service," *Milbank Memorial Fund Quarterly/Health and Society* 57 (Winter 1979): 70-94.
20. H. F. Pitkin, *The Concept of Representation* (Berkeley: University of California Press, 1967), p. 3.
21. T. R. Marmor, "Consumer Representation: Beneath the Consensus, Many Difficulties," *Trustee* 30 (1977): 37-40.
22. H. F. Pitkin, *The Concept of Representation,* p. 8.
23. A. P. Griffiths, "How Can One Person Represent Another?" *Aristotelian Society,* Suppl. Vol. 34 (1960): 187-208.
24. H. F. Pitkin, *The Concept of Representation.*
25. A. Birch, *Representation* (New York: Praeger, 1971), p. 20.
26. M. C. Swabey, "The Representative Sample", in H. F. Pitkin, *Representation* (New York: Atherton, 1969): C. J. Friedrich, *Constitutional Government and Democracy* (New York: Blaisdell, 1950), pp. 266ff.
27. H. F. Pitkin, *The Concept of Representation,* p. 60.
28. For notable formulations of this common idea, see Edmund Burke, "The English Constitutional System," in Pitkin (1969); or James Madison, "The Problem of Faction in a Republic," in *The Federalist* (New York: Modern Library, 1937).
29. J. D. Greenstone and P. E. Peterson, *Race and Authority in Urban Politics: Consumer Participation and the War on Poverty* (Chicago: University of Chicago Press, 1973), Chapter 6.
30. B. Barry, *Political Argument* (London: Routledge & Kegan Paul, 1965), Chapter 10; I. Balbus, "The Concept of Interest in Pluralist and Marxian Analysis," in I. Katznelson, et al., eds, *The Politics and Society Reader* (New York: David McKay, 1972); R. Flatham, *The Public Interest* (New York: John Wiley, 1966).
31. M. Edelman, *The Symbolic Use of Politics* (Urbana: University of Illinois Press, 1967); H. F. Pitkin, ed., *Representation* (New York: Atherton, 1969), Chapter 10.
32. Greenstone and Peterson, *Race and Authority.*
33. Codman Research Group, "The Impact of Health Planning and Regulation on the Patterns of Hospital Utilization in New England," Executive Summary, DHEW Contract 291-76-0003, Final Report, Year 1, September, 1977.
34. W. Clark, "Placebo or Cure?" p. 55.
35. P. C. Schmitter, *An Inventory of Analytical Pluralist Propositions,* unpublished monograph, University of Chicago, 1975.
36. J. M. Berry, *Lobbying for the People* (Princeton, NJ: Princeton University Press, 1977); M. U. Nadel, *The Politics of Consumer Protection* (Indianapolis: Bobbs-Merrill, 1971); A. McFarland, *Public Interest Lobbies* (Washington, DC: American Enterprise Institute, 1976).
37. Greenstone and Peterson, *Race and Authority.*
38. M. Lipsky and M. Lounds, "Citizen Participation and Health Care: Problems of Government Induced Participation," *Journal of Health Politics, Policy and Law* 1 (Spring 1976): 107.

39. PL 93-641, §(b)(3)(C)(iii)(II).

40. PL 93-641, §1512(b)(3)(C)(i).

41. For a similar list, see Georgia Legal Services Program, "Proposed Amendments to PL 93-641," December 9, 1977, #3. To avoid litigation, regulations should make clear that this is a residual category to be filled at the discretion of the secretary, not a sweeping general provision mandating representation slots for all identifiable groups having significant health care interests.

42. J. D. Greenstone, *Group Theories,* p. 244.

43. C. Anderson, "Political Design and the Representation of Interests," *Comparative Political Studies* 10 (April 1977).

44. T. R. Marmor and A. Bridges, "Comparative Policy Analysis and Health Planning Processes Internationally," prepared for the director of the Bureau of Health Planning and Resources Development, DHEW, May 1977; revised for *Journal of Health Politics, Policy, and Law,* forthcoming.

45. T. R. Marmor, "Welfare Medicine: How Success Can Be a Failure," *Yale Law Journal* 85 (July 1976).

46. V. Sidel and R. Sidel, *A Healthy State* (New York: Pantheon, 1977).

47. L. Hartz, *The Liberal Tradition in America* (New York: Harcourt Brace Jovanovich, 1955); A. Shonfield, *Modern Capitalism* (New York: Oxford University Press, 1965).

48. M. Friedman, *Capitalism and Freedom* (Chicago: University of Chicago Press, 1962); F. Hayek, *The Road to Serfdom* (Chicago: University of Chicago Press, 1944); L. Von Mises, *Liberalism and Socio-Economic Exposition* (Kansas City: Sheed, Andrews & McMeel, 1962).

49. C. E. Lindblom, "The Science of Muddling Through," *Public Administration Review* 19 (Spring 1959).

50. Inglehart, "Health Report: State, County Governments Win Key Roles in New Program," *National Journal* (November 8, 1973).

51. J. Sundquist and D. Davis, *Making Federalism Work* (Washington, DC: Brookings, 1969), p. 7.

52. R. Hudson, "A Bloc Grant to the States for Long Term Care," University Health Policy Consortium, Waltham, Massachusetts, February 2, 1979.

53. S. Beer, "Federalism, Nationalism and Democracy in America," *American Political Science Review* 72 (March 1978).

54. See, for example, the report by the Committee on Interstate Commerce and Foreign Commerce on the National Health Policy, Planning and Resources Development Act of 1974. Report No. 93-1382, Washington, D.C., Government Printing Office, November 26, 1974.

55. G. McConnell, *Private Power;* F. Taylor, "Scientific Management," in D. J. Pugh, ed., *Organizational Theory* (New York: Penguin, 1971.)

56. *Business Week* 6 August 1979: 54.

57. A. McFarland, "'Third Forces' in American Politics: The Case of Common Cause," in J. Fishel, ed., *Parties and Elections in an Anti-Party Age* (Bloomington: University of Indiana Press, 1978).

Chapter 9

Future Policy Directions
The Political Economy of Competition

In this book we argue for realistic evaluation and comparison of public policy alternatives for American medicine. We reject the naive view that the private market for medical care is entirely self-regulating. But we also question the equally naive argument that the identification of actual or potential market failure is a sufficient condition for further government intervention. The political process is clearly flawed as a mechanism for correcting market "wrongs," whatever their origin. While in some cases, intervention may yield results that unambiguously improve market outcomes, in other instances public policy may increase dysfunction in the medical care delivery system. In evaluating public policy proposals, the limitations of government should be acknowledged just as systematically as the limitations of market processes. This suggests a synthesis of the traditional roles of economists and the political scientists.

Over the past twenty years, the traditional boundaries between economics and political science *have* gradually faded (explaining in part the collaboration of the authors of this book), and a "political-economic" approach to policy analysis has emerged. This model emphasizes the conflicting motives of politicians and bureaucrats, and the uncertain and biased information available to them. Since the "public interest" cannot be precisely defined, they must balance pressures from numerous groups with conflicting interests and with varying degrees of ability to pursue those interests. Therefore, the outcomes of political or regulatory processes in medical care are likely to depend primarily on the number of gainers and losers associated with a given policy proposal, the relative magnitudes of the gains and losses, and the ability of the affected groups to organize and participate in the political process. A knowledge of these factors will contribute more toward an understanding of observed medical care policy than will evaluation of the contribution of a particular policy proposal to the "economic efficiency" of the medical care system.

The analysis of the previous chapters applies this basic premise in five different policy areas. In Chapter 4, Marmor, Wittman, and Heagy discuss the potential for bold government action to control medical care inflation. They point to an "imbalanced political market" as reason for the rejection of theoretically sound methods for inflation control proposed by economists. In their view, doctors, hospital administrators, union officials, and insurers will oppose all potentially successful policies to restrain inflation, since the costs of such policies are concentrated on them. They likely will be successful; the benefits from inflation control are diffused among all consumers, leaving few rewards for the politician who supports efforts to control medical inflation. In fact, the greater the likely effectiveness of proposals to introduce market restraints on medical inflation, the greater the opposition of concentrated interests, and the less likely it becomes that such policies will be implemented. The authors conclude that, "in the absence of some concentrated interest, the political market is unlikely to adopt a policy simply because it constitutes a public good."

In their analysis of the political economy of national health insurance, Bowler, Kudrle, and Marmor describe the political marketplace for this policy as quite complex. This is because the redistribution of income, influence, and status, and the legitimacy of highly valued political beliefs, and symbols, are at stake. National health insurance is traditionally favored by unions and a loose coalition of "liberals and consumers," but opposed by physicians, hospitals, insurance companies, and a weak coalition of conservative and business groups. Because of this relatively balanced political marketplace, the authors (writing in 1977) accurately observed that "enactment of NHI legislation in the near future is not inevitable" and predicted that it is not even likely with strong and energetic presidential leadership. National health insurance was not a high priority in the Carter Administration and has not subsequently been enacted, despite earlier pronouncements by some policy analysts concerning its inevitability.

In Chapter 6, Christianson and McClure assess the prospects for reduction of excess hospital capacity through public sector actions. They identify several failures in the political marketplace which can lead to an overemphasis on direct, "command-and-control" strategies for reducing hospital capacity when indirect, incentive-oriented approaches could prove more efficient. However, the relative unattractiveness of incentive-altering strategies as political goods (a feature noted by Marmor, Wittman, and Heagy as well) means their implementation would be difficult. Recognizing this fact, Christianson and McClure offer a sequenced implementation strategy designed to offset, in part, the political limitations of incentive strategies.

In Chapter 7, Christianson analyzes the regulatory process in long-term care using the "political-economic" model. He develops a theory of enforcement, based on the self-interest of bureaucrats, which emphasizes the limited nature of available information and the conflicting pressures imposed on the regulatory process by legislators, other agencies, and special interest groups. He concludes that the historical record of incomplete enforcement of long-term care regulations is consistent with this theory, and that enforcement is not likely to improve until a policy is devised which alters the presently imbalanced political marketplace in long-term care.

Finally, in Chapter 8, Marmor and Morone examine the problem of obtaining representative consumer participation in health planning. They argue that "narrow, concentrated producer interests are more likely to pay the costs of political action than broad, diffuse, consumer interests." Furthermore, producer groups have the advantage of ongoing organizations and possess information and expertise that are essential to the health planning process. Their interest in health planning decisions is constant, while the interest of consumers is intermittent and likely to be focused on specific issues. For all of these reasons, it is difficult to obtain effective, ongoing consumer representation in health planning. In order to enhance the potential for effective representation, Marmor and Morone propose (1) that some health planning staff be assigned directly to consumers, and (2) that planning-board members be chosen as direct representatives of interest groups. These suggestions would increase the amount of information and expertise available to consumers while also making consumer representatives directly accountable to well-defined constituencies. In this way some of the imbalance in the health planning process currently favoring producers might be corrected.

These five chapters, in presenting specific applications of the political-economic model, illustrate the usefulness of the model in understanding a variety of medical care policies. They also demonstrate the utility of the approach in going beyond analysis of past policy disappointments. The political-economic approach is also useful in improving the design of policy proposals and evaluating the likelihood that specific policy initiatives will be enacted. It is in the latter spirit that we conclude this book with a brief analysis of the political potential for the "competitive strategy," a set of proposals that apparently will receive considerable attention by health policymakers in the 1980s.

The Competitive Strategy: The Future for Medical Care Policy?

As a long-run approach to medical care delivery system reform, and particularly to the restraint of medical care expenditure increases, several officials in the Reagan Administration—including HHS Secretary Schweiker and Budget Director Stockman—have publicly supported a set of ideas known as the "competitive strategy." The basic premise of the competitive strategy, as developed by Enthoven, McClure, Havighurst, Ellwood, and others (see Chapter 1), is that the present medical care system contains little reward for consumers who choose efficient providers or for providers who are cost-effective in their practice of medicine. According to these advocates, this lack of cost-conscious incentives is primarily due to the prevalence of comprehensive third-party insurance. For example, whether an individual enters the most expensive hospital or the lowest-cost hospital, insurance is likely to pay most of the cost and the insurance premium will not be affected preceptibly by the choice. When providers order fewer services for their patients (even though fewer services may be appropriate), their income suffers, since the existing reimbursement system pays them less; their efficiency is irrelevant and even invisible to consumers.

Advocates of the competitive strategy believe that restructuring these incentives is crucial to the restraint of medical care expenditure increases, and consequently public expenditures for medical care, in the long run. They argue that the key to revising the present incentives is the introduction of greater price competition in the delivery of medical care. Competition could develop over fees and charges if substantial consumer cost-sharing were introduced in present insurance policies. However, the political prospects for "rolling back" present comprehensive third-party insurance coverage on a large scale seem poor. Therefore, assuming that comprehensive insurance remains widespread, price competition must center on premiums.

Premium competition could be established by creating sets of providers who compete with each other and with conventional providers and insurers on the basis of services, coverage, and premiums under neutral market conditions. These provider groupings are sometimes called "health care plans," to distinguish them from the more narrowly defined health maintenance organizations (see Chapter 6). Each plan could be organized in a variety of ways. They could accommodate most existing practice arrangements, including solo practice and fee for service reimbursement, with minimal modification. The most important feature of the plans in stimulating competition is that they distinguish between specific sets of physicians and hospitals, with a separate premium for each. The consumer choosing the most efficient set of providers is rewarded by a lower premium and/or greater benefits. Attractive and efficient providers are rewarded by enrollment growth, thereby creating incentives for cost-consciousness on the part of providers and consumers. Low-income individuals presumably would have access to this market through medical vouchers that would play a role analogous to food stamps or housing subsides.

In addition to stimulating the formation of health care plans, the competitive strategy would attempt to create market conditions under which these plans could compete on an equal footing with existing insurance plans. Typical "rules of the game" proposed by some advocates of the competitive strategy include:

(1) Relatively few barriers to the formation of new health care plans,
(2) A requirement that no plan could contain all providers in a given area,
(3) Freedom for consumers to choose among plans, which translates into a requirement (or recommendation) that benefit programs, such as those offered by private employers and Medicare, provide consumers with a multiple choice of health care and insurance plans,
(4) Freedom for plans to compete by offering different combinations of benefits, premiums and service levels, and
(5) A requirement (or inducement) for employers or government to pay a fixed amount that could be applied toward any health benefit option, with the consumer paying, or being rebated, the balance, thus creating a reward for consumers who choose cost-effective providers.

To date, the legislative proposals pertaining to the competitive strategy have focused primarily on establishing these competitive market conditions, rather than on the stimulation of new plans. For instance, Senator Durenberger's Health Incentive Reform Act of 1979 would require all employers in organizations above a certain size to offer employees a choice of health plans, with a fixed dollar contribution to whichever plan was chosen. Tax deductibility of employer contributions would be limited to some predetermined amount to be adjusted annually. Furthermore Medicare beneficiaries would be permitted to direct that an amount equal to their "adjusted average per capita cost" to Medicare be paid to a health care plan as a fixed prospective premium contribution. Other bills have advocated similar options for Medicaid beneficiaries. While most bills have contained these types of "market entry" provisions, there seems to be a disagreement among competition advocates concerning the desirable level of government involvement in the formation of new health care plans. Some argue that opening up the market to health care plans would provide sufficient stimulus for the development of a substantial number of new plans. Others contend that government loans are required to induce providers to form health care plans given the historical opposition of organized medicine to any type of prepaid plan. Competitive advocates also disagree over the desirability of proscribing a minimum benefit package for health care plans. Enthoven argues that this is necessary to make consumer choices less complex and to ensure that minimum inpatient coverage is provided in all plans. On the other hand, Stockman believes that this would lead to excessive pleading by special interests groups which Congress would be unable to resist. Consequently, he favors no minimum benefit requirements.[1]

Regardless of their positions on particular legislative proposals, supporters of the competitive strategy seem to feel that the Reagan Administration provides an environment conducive to its implementation. For instance, Alain Enthoven notes that, "philosophically, President-elect Reagan and his supporters are more comfortable with an approach to cost control based on incentives in a decentralized market than their predecessors were. Thus it should not be surprising that the

'Report of the Chairman of the Health Policy Advisory Group' to President-elect Ronald Reagan recommended giving first priority to the development of a compromise version of the various pro-competitive bills that can be broadly supported."[2]

As in the debate over national health insurance conducted in the 1970s, the competitive strategy "raises familiar ideological charges and counter charges, symbols and slogans" relating to the appropriate role of government in the delivery of medical care (Chapter 5). Unlike national health insurance, a successful competitive strategy presumably would reduce the long-run involvement of government in the medical care system. Also, it seems unlikely that "the national political party and interest group alignments associated with these symbols and with the broad issue of government's role in the economy" (Chapter 5) will coalesce along the traditional lines that characterized the national health insurance debate. The powerful, organized provider interest groups that opposed national health insurance, partially on the grounds that it would increase the role of government, will not necessarily support the competitive strategy because it promises to reduce government's role. In fact, a closer examination of the characteristics of incentive-based strategies in the political process in general and the objectives and past actions of organized medical interest groups in particular suggests that the enactment of procompetitive legislation under the Reagan Administration is highly uncertain. Paradoxically, it can be argued that comprehensive procompetitive legislation would have a greater chance of enactment during a Democratic administration.

An important impediment to the enactment of pro-competitive legislation is the indirect relationship between an effective competitive market and reductions in medical care expenditures, and particularly those expenditures that are part of the federal budget. Just as there does not appear to be any regulatory "quick fix" to expenditure increases for medical care, the competitive strategy also would not produce immediate visible gains. Even its most optimistic supporters acknowledge that it probably would take ten to fifteen years for a competitive market to develop and, if effective, to begin to reduce medical care expenditures in any given area. During this development period, medical care expenditures would continue to increase, as would pressures on politicians to "do something." It is even possible that the early stages of competition could accelerate the rate of increase in total community medical care expenditures if traditional providers react to the loss of patients by increasing fees or utilization. Although this provider strategy would ultimately increase insurance rates and drive more consumers into health care plans, it would temporarily contribute to rising medical care expenditures. Thus, the competitive strategy does not promise the quick, visible results desired by politicians in their reelection efforts.

Furthermore, the eventual outcome of a competitive strategy in uncertain, since it has never before been implemented on a wide scale. There are some initially promising results emerging from communities such as Minneapolis-St. Paul,[3] but competition is in the embryonic stage even in the Twin Cities. Therefore, there is no strong empirical evidence to support theoretical predictions concerning the long-term benefits of the competitive strategy. While these benefits may indeed occur, their uncertain potential may not be sufficient to capture the support of the typically risk-averse politician.

Finally, it would be difficult to determine the relative effectiveness of the competitive strategy, even should the rate of increase in medical care expenditures eventually decline. There will be many natural changes in the medical care delivery system over the next ten years, irrespective of the actions government might take to promote competition. In addition, other government policies relating to medical care will be adopted during this same period. Therefore it would be difficult to isolate the ultimate impact on medical care expenditures of incentive-changing, competitive policies, even should they prove to be successful. For all of these reasons, the potential political "benefits" accruing to politicians for support of the competitive strategy, even if it succeeds in reducing the rate of medical care expenditure increase, are not compelling.

These general considerations suggest that the competitive strategy is not a particularly attractive political good for the vote-maximizing politician. An examination of the groups that stand to gain and to lose if the competitive strategy proves effective supports this conclusion. Clearly, the general voting public would gain from an effective competitive strategy to the extent that it reduced increases in their taxes, insurance, and medical service payments. However, these benefits are likely to be small individually, hard to identify, and even harder to associate with the relatively subtle changes advocated by the competitive approach. Politicians are not likely to enact pro-competitive legislation because of the political support to be gained from the general public.

Employers constitute a second benefiting group, since they are major purchasers of health services through their contributions toward the premiums of employee health benefit options. To the extent that competition promises to be effective, it seems logical that employers would support the strategy. However, in most cases an employer who acts individually to offer a multiple benefit choice with a fixed premium contribution realizes no immediate savings from the action and will have only a negligible impact on the development of competition in any given community. A majority of community employers must decide to take these actions if an effective market is to be developed. The desirability of joint action by employers provides the justification for the pro-competitive legislation mentioned previously. But, from the employer's perspective, this proposed pro-competitive legislation is not costless. It reduces the employer's freedom to limit the number of benefit options for employees and to negotiate with employees over contributions; it also may increase the costs of administration of health benefits. Employers who are self-insured could find the cost savings from self-insurance eroded if substantial numbers of employees chose competing health care plans. Therefore, active employer support for the competitive strategy may be difficult to sustain.

A third benefiting group consists of government agencies with an interest in protecting their own budgets by reducing the expenditures of the Health Care Financing Administration. These agencies might support efforts to extend the competitive model to program beneficiaries as a cost-reducing measure. However, it seems more likely that they would advocate lids on these program expenditures and/or benefit restrictions as more effective, immediate methods of accomplishing the same objectives.

Even though the competitive strategy may not be a particularly attractive proposal in a general political sense, the Reagan Administration nevertheless might support its implementation for purely philosophical reasons, providing that the potential for political losses is small. The primary losers from any effective reduction in the rate of increase in medical expenditures are medical care providers (see Chapter 4). It is interesting to observe that provider organizations did not actively oppose the competitive strategy during the Carter Administration; in fact, some provider groups indicated support for it. At that time they perceived the likely alternative as increased, more comprehensive, regulation. In this environment, the competitive strategy seemed the lesser to two evils. Under the Reagan Administration, increased regulation is now a highly unlikely alternative and the initial enthusiasm of some provider organizations for the competitive strategy has waned as a consequence. Most provider groups now support the "deregulation" aspects of David Stockman's National Health Care Reform Act of 1980, which would eliminate federal health planning and PSRO legislation, but some are changing their positions on those features of other legislative proposals that would create competitive market conditions. The Federation of American Hospitals, the national lobby of the proprietary hospital management companies, remains an aggressive supporter of the competitive approach. However, the views of the American Medical Association and the American Hospital Association are now in flux. As Iglehart observes, "it's fair to say that many of their members have strong reservations about how competition would impact on their pocketbooks and their operations."[4] He also notes that these organizations "formed the basis of a strong private sector effort which led to the demise of the Carter administration's hospital cost containment bill."[5]

Since private medical care lobbies, and the American Medical Association in particular, have traditionally been strong supporters of the Republican party, one would expect their influence to be greater in the Reagan Administration than under a Democratic president. There is some historical evidence to support this conjecture; the American Medical Association played a prominent role in the emasculation of the Health Maintenance Strategy of 1970, the less sophisticated, but in many ways more ambitious, intellectual predecessor of the competitive strategy. As described by Falkson, the Medical Association's effort was two-tiered: public support for the HMO concept (while taking every opportunity to point out faults) combined with intensive private lobbying efforts to kill the legislation. These private efforts appear to have been extremely effective in causing the Nixon Administration drastically to reduce its commitment to the HMO program.[6] One can easily conceive of a similar professional association strategy with respect to competitive reforms: public support for the selective deregulation of medical care and the virtues of private enterprise combined with private lobbying efforts to kill any legislation that would lead to effective price competition through a restructuring of the current delivery system.

In this scenario, if the Reagan Administration vigorously pursues pro-competitive legislation on ideological grounds, it risks the loss of traditional Republican sources of political support and campaign funding. The political solution is to continue to extol the virtues of deregulation, publicly support the desirability of price-sensitive competition, but fail to pursue the reforms in the medical care marketplace which are essential if this competition is to take place. Legislation would be limited to opening the Medicare market for easier access by health care plans, provided that immediate savings in federal monies could be realized; or it would emphasize the desirability of limiting the tax deductibility of health care premiums as a means of generating additional tax revenue for the Administration's budget balancing efforts.

A failure to enact legislation in support of the competitive strategy would not necessarily spell its doom. As pointed out in Chapter 6, experience with government legislation of incentive-based policies in general, and with HMOs in particular, suggests that it has not been especially effective. There is no reason to believe that new pro-competitive legislation would be an exception in this regard. Therefore, the competitive strategy might be well served by the scenario we have presented: educational effort and public support from the Reagan Administration, but very little legislation. This could result in the gradual development of increased competition in communities that are receptive to it, preserve the freedom for new methods of medical care delivery to develop without legislated restrictions, and permit careful assessment of the outcomes of competitive markets where they do occur.

NOTES

1. John K. Iglehart, "Washington Report," *Journal of Health Politics,* Policy and Law 6 (Summer 1981): 362-363.
2. Alain C. Enthoven, "The Competition Strategy: Status and Prospects," *New England Journal of Medicine* 304 (January 8, 1981): 111.
3. Jon B. Christianson and Walter McClure, "Competition in the Delivery of Medical Care," *New England Journal of Medicine* 301 (October 11, 1979): 812-818.
4. Iglehart, "Washington Report," p. 364.
5. Ibid.
6. Joseph L. Falkson, *HMOs and the Politics of Health System Reform* (Chicago: American Hospital Association, 1980), pp. 145-146.

About the Authors

THEODORE R. MARMOR received his A.B. and Ph.D. degrees from Harvard, held research fellowships at Wadham and Nuffield Colleges, Oxford, and taught at the Universities of Minnesota, Wisconsin, Essex (England), and Chicago before joining Yale's faculty as Professor of Political Science and Public Health and Chairman of the Center for Health Studies. He has authored *The Politics of Medicare* and numerous articles on the politics and policies of the welfare state, particularly emphasizing social security, national health insurance, and health planning. He is an editor of and contributor to *National Health Insurance: Conflicting Goals and Policy Choices.* Mr. Marmor became the editor of the *Journal of Health Politics, Policy and Law* in summer 1980. He was special assistant to HEW's undersecretary in 1966, was on the staff of the President's Commission on Income Maintenance Programs (1968-1970), and served on the recent Presidential Commission on a National Agenda for the eighties.

JON B. CHRISTIANSON is Associate Professor of Public Policy, Planning and Administration and Associate Professor of Economics at the University of Arizona in Tucson, where he is also a faculty participant in the Health Care Management Program. He received a Ph.D. in economics from the University of Wisconsin, Madison, in 1974. Since that time his research interests have included the application of cost-benefit techniques to medical care evaluation, the regulation of long-term care, economic issues relating to rural health care delivery, community care alternatives to nursing homes, health maintenance organizations, and competitive approaches to reform of the medical care system. He has published in these areas in numerous professional journals and serves often as a consultant to federal and state government agencies and legislators.